'Dr Wright has written a remarkable book. She organisation is fundamental to structuring experience. Outside and inside the consulting room, outside and inside the transference. She bases her profound theory on diverse sources, including Freud's many drawings, and extensive clinical experience. Her ideas on spatialisation will generate new areas of investigation and practice and will evoke a eureka recognition of the unconscious ordering of everyday life.'

Karl Figlio, *Clinical Associate, British Psychoanalytical Society*
Professor Emeritus, University of Essex, UK

'Deborah Wright shows us an interesting and somewhat hidden tradition from Freud onwards. The consulting room and indeed all living spaces are given individual meanings by each of us, depending on our individual and cultural experiences. Our Unconscious 'space' offers a necessary dimension in addition to the transference to the person of the therapist who inhabits the space. The author provides clinical evidence, as well as cultural, to show how it can be exposed and used.'

Dr. R.D. Hinshelwood, *Psychoanalyst, and Professor*
Emeritus, University of Essex, UK

'It is a truth universally acknowledged in psychoanalytic/psychody-namic discourse that the consulting room or 'setting', in which clinical work takes place, is of particular importance. Why that should be, beyond what seems 'obvious', however is under-theorised in the literature. Dr Wright rectifies this in her scholarly and accessible book in which she presents clinical observation which advances current theory and practice. She formulates a clear language and terminology to articulate her theory of spatial dynamics, and her own uncanny illustrations add depth to her discourse. The book is a delight to read and essential for teaching and training purposes.'

Meg Errington, *Psychoanalytic Psychotherapist*
British Psychoanalytic Council, UK

The Physical and Virtual Space of the Consulting Room

In this thought-provoking book, Deborah Wright examines the role of both space and objects as they become manifest in the psychoanalytic process and looks at how the role of the consulting room in the therapeutic process is both primitive and transferential.

Wright explores spatialisation as simultaneously being a psychological projection of meaning and as physically acting upon the environment, utilised to master the undifferentiated, relentless, internal pressure of instinct. Throughout *The Physical and Virtual Space of the Consulting Room*, she considers the spatial aspects of work with patients by foregrounding the importance of the consulting room and its contents, including the impact of changes of consulting room, travelling, and in working virtually. Illustrated with clinical material and hand-drawn artwork, Wright orients the reader in the new territory by going beyond the existing literature that considers the objects and space of the consulting room solely as transferential aspects of the analyst.

The interdisciplinary approach in this book calls on psychoanalytic theory and technique as well as philosophy, history, archaeology, and anthropology, which will be of great interest to all psychoanalytically orientated therapists as well as anyone, clinical or non-clinical, who makes use of psychoanalysis.

Dr Deborah L. S. Wright, D.Psychodyn.Psych, BPC MBACP FPC, is a Psychotherapist in private practice and an Academic, Lecturer, and Programme Director of the Clinical Professional Doctorate Programs, in the Department of Psychosocial and Psychoanalytic Studies at The University of Essex, as well as an Artist, Printmaker, and Illustrator.

The Physical and Virtual Space of the Consulting Room

Room-object Spaces

Deborah L. S. Wright

Routledge
Taylor & Francis Group

LONDON AND NEW YORK

Cover image: © Deborah L. S. Wright

First published 2022
by Routledge
4 Park Square, Milton Park, Abingdon, Oxon OX14 4RN

and by Routledge
605 Third Avenue, New York, NY 10158

Routledge is an imprint of the Taylor & Francis Group, an informa business

British Library Cataloguing-in-Publication Data
A catalogue record for this book is available from the British Library

Library of Congress Cataloguing-in-Publication Data
A catalog record has been requested for this book

ISBN: 978-1-032-02875-0 (hbk)
ISBN: 978-1-032-03595-6 (pbk)
ISBN: 978-1-003-18811-7 (ebk)

DOI: 10.4324/9781003188117

Typeset in Times New Roman
by MPS Limited, Dehradun

To my son John and Mum; Always there

Contents

Figures

Acknowledgements

I wish to thank Professor Karl Figlio, for his invaluable thinking-with-space, Professor Bob Hinshelwood and Professor Sue Kegerreis for always challenging and pushing my thinking and Meg Errington, for all her containing thinking. I wish to thank Ellie Duncan and Jana Craddock at Routledge for her always kind and generous help with all processes. All of the University of Essex, Department of Psychosocial and Psychoanalytic Studies staff and academics who supported this project, in particular Dr Chris Nicholson for so much enthusiasm and Alison Evans whose thoughtful help and knowledge has been invaluable. Also, in the University of Essex library Special Collections, Sandy and Lucy for all of their help with finding Freud's letters. I want to thank Chris Stringer, at the Natural History Museum, for conversations and thoughts on the latest global findings on Neanderthal spaces. I wish to thank Saliann St-Clair at The Marsh Agency for all her great help and the Marsh Agency for permission to use Sigmund Freud's drawings. To Bryony Davies at the Freud Museum for always being so helpful and good at finding things as well as the Freud Museum for permission to use images. And I wish to thank Palgrave for permission to use extracts from my book chapters. And to thank my Mum, who supported this research from the beginning and would have loved to see this manifestation of it. Alastair and John for all their unending support and Julie Nicholson for being there.

Chapter 1

Introduction and Background: Spatialisation in Spaces and Rooms

[This chapter contains material from

the book Chapter; Wright, D. (2018) 'Rooms as Replacements for People: The Consulting Room as a Room Object' (pp. 251–262) in 'Psychoanalysis' section of 'On Replacement – Cultural, Social and Psychological Representations', Eds: Jean Owen and Naomi Segal, Switzerland, Palgrave Macmillan.

And; Wright, D. (2019) 'Spatialisation and the Fomenting of Political Violence' (pp. 167–187) in Fomenting Political Violence – Fantasy, Language, Media, Action.', Eds. Steffen Kruger, Karl Figlio, Barry Richards. Switzerland, Palgrave Macmillan. Reproduced with permission of Palgrave Macmillan.]

Introduction

This book began with a study, shown in Chapter 4, originating from my observation of phenomena relating to patients' relationships with the consulting room, where they project into the room, at times seemingly unrelated to the transference to me. Current theories do not completely address this, including an assumption that for the patient everything in the room is related to the transference. I consider that the role of the consulting room in the therapeutic process is both primitive (pre-transferential) and transferential and my discovery is that the former has not been noted before and the latter has not been adequately understood. Sigmund Freud invented the psychoanalytic consulting room as well as the concept of transference. However, despite his fascination with spatiality, and, as I show in his work, his projection of maternal and paternal figures into room spaces, including his consulting room, this remains untheorized. In addition, Freud made spatial diagrams to illustrate his theoretical concepts and many of those concepts have an implicit spatial concern. A neglected area of Psychoanalysis is the extent to which Freud was interested in space and objects to understand the psyche and also the psychoanalytic process in the consulting room.

DOI: 10.4324/9781003188117-1

Freud was deeply immersed in spatiality in culture but this has not received much attention in literature. My formulation of spatialisation simultaneously involves a psychological projection of meaning and physically acting upon the environment, utilised to master the undifferentiated, relentless, internal pressure of instinct. I suggest that spatialisation is a distinctive feature of mental life and therapeutic work. Spatialisation is part of normal development and people retreat into it when under stress or when they are insecure. I suggest that the less thinking takes place, the more spatialising happens. Richard Wollheim (1969) wrote that in the mind's primitive state thoughts become, as I suggest, spatial, and they are projected outward as a way of dealing with the emotions so that instead of thinking actions occur in space. Linked directly with Freud's theory of projection this means that thinking primitively means thinking spatially. Object-relations theory is inadequate without spatialisation in that Object-relations are dimensional. It fits with it, and does not replace Object-relations theories; it adds another aspect, the spatialised aspect. The Room-object Spatial Matrix offers a missing way of understanding people's relationship with the consulting room. A fundamental feature of Object-relations is transference, transference is built on spatialisation, spatialisation is the foundation of mental functioning. You don't have an object to transfer until you have spatialisation. There is no object without spatialisation, Spatialising - leads to - Object-relations - leads to - transference. The more primitive the levels of mental functioning, the more spatial it is. I am now going to analyse spatialisation in this study.

I utilise Freud's theory of instinct (1915, p. 120) as being unformed internal pressure of instinct put into spatial form, as well as; historical and cultural examples of space use and spatialising examples (here in Chapter 1); Sigmund Freud's writings and diagrams of spatial usage and spatialising (in Chapter 2), as well the perspectives of Richard Wollheim on thinking and Object Relations and Winnicottian theories (in Chapter 3) to formulate my hypothetical addition to the theory of transference to explain the phenomena better: The Room-object Spatial Matrix. I suggest that this can take place within a matrix of stages, the first of which, *Primal Spatialisation*, takes place into mother/parts of mother to create the object, this is pre-object and therefore pre-transferential. I suggest that a difficulty in utilising mother as the first object of spatialisation, can lead to *Stage 2* of the Matrix, *Room-object*, where spatialising into the spatial array of room spaces and the objects within them replaces or supplements the mother function, topping up the object usage of parts of mother including the insides and parts of the insides of mother, the outsides of mother and parts thereof, including mothers skin, which can be spatialised in the outside and inside of the room walls and room contents. *Stage 3 – Consulting Room-object*, is where the consulting room is used as other rooms were used before as a direct displacement from one room to the other separate from transference to the therapist. *Stage 4 – Consulting Room-object + Transference*, is like stage 3 but includes the transference to the therapist. *Stage 5 – Consulting Room-object + Transference, outside the Consulting room,* includes the spatialising of original spatialised room, the object, the therapist in the transference and the therapist's consulting room. These stages can be moved in and out of, the stages representing a regressive, defensive function (re-enacting the spatialising to re-create the object and defend against its loss), as well as a maturational one as a form of rudimentary containing mind. I suggest that spatialised room transference into rooms (Room-objects) can fulfil the role of an external auxiliary thinking/mind space as a replacement for and an addition to mother's or, in the case of the consulting room, the therapist's containing mind. My claim is that part of this hypothetical Room-object Spatial Matrix is pre-object and therefore pre-transferential. My methodology in the original study (shown in Chapter 4), was an attempt to magnify the primitive spatial level of thinking. I utilise clinical material in Chapter 4, from this study, relating to room moves, to demonstrate where the formulation of the Room-object Spatial Matrix stages can and cannot be seen, in order to demonstrate the matrix stages, in particular the pre-transferential aspects. In Chapter 5 there is a discussion of findings of the clinical study and implications for practice.

In Chapter 6 on The Room-object Spatial Matrix in the Virtual consulting room space, I show clinical work relating to a different room move; one to the Virtual consulting room, relating to the Covid-19 pandemic. This was also a global room move, creating the greatest spatial change on masse relating to the psychotherapy consulting room space, since Sigmund Freud first created it (as discussed in Chapter 2) and heralding, for all therapists (including those who had not worked virtually beforehand), a new potentially 'blended delivery' and we could say 'blended rooms' (physical and virtual) psychotherapy age. I explore patients' spatialising activities in the virtual Consulting room and their attempts at the *Stage 5 – Consulting Room-object + Transference, outside the Consulting room,* having had to be creative in their spatialising outside the consulting room space; forming their own couchs, chairs, and spaces. For those who have never been in the physical consulting room space, they have also been able to utilise parts of the virtual space to formulate the *Stage 5*, something of which is necessitated in the Virtual consulting room space as patients. Whether patients have been in a physical consulting room space or not, they have had to make something of a room space to create a room for themselves to do the psychotherapy work in, to be part of the virtual consulting room. This chapter looks beyond the Consulting Room at psychosocial applications of the Room-object Spatial Matrix to the novels of E.M. Forster. Forster's language of expression is spatial, concerning people's relationships to the interiors of rooms, spaces, houses, street, cities, and countryside, including colonial, post-colonial, capitalist (pre-neoliberal), and queer perspective spaces, often as a spatialisation. This chapter also considers both the social themes he explored in his novels and the rooms and spaces within them and how applying the Room-object Spatial Matrix can bring out psychosocial thinking on these themes and spaces allowing for an additional layer to be considered. The final end Chapter, Chapter 9, concerns endings and goes backwards through the chapters of the book looking at clinical examples, Freud's room spaces, and cultural examples back to the beginning. It concerns people's final rooms in which they spend their final days, which I suggest can be thought of as an additional stage of the Room-object Spatial Matrix; *Stage 6 – The End Room-object* space. I include a clinical example, with that of Andre Gide's mother and Sigmund Freud's own *End Room-object* space; his consulting room, including the last book he was reading at the end in that space, Balzac's 'La Peau de Chagrin', where the magic skin on the wall is reminiscent of the *Room-object* and its illustration in Chapter 3, of the walls as mother's skin. Beyond the Room-object Spatial Matrix I suggest that there are *Post Room-object* spaces exemplified by examples from Westminster Abbey, which are first discussed here in Chapter 1. Finally, there are conclusions on the physical and virtual consulting room space in relation to the Room-object spatial matrix and implications for practice through the book.

Background and Rationale for Formulation of the Room-object Spatial Matrix: Spatial Thinking in the Psychoanalytic Discipline, in Particular Concerning the Consulting Room

As part of the background and rationale for my formulation of the Room-object spatial matrix, I will now look at spatial thinking applied to the psychoanalytic discipline, in particular concerning the consulting room. Robert Tally discussed Michel Foucault's characterisation of this 'epoch of space':

> As Foucault announced, '[t]he great obsession of the nineteenth century was, as we know, history: with its themes of development and suspension, of crisis, and cycle [...]. The present epoch will perhaps be above all the epoch of space. We are in the epoch of simultaneity: we are in the epoch of juxtaposition, the epoch of the near and far, of the side-by-side, [...] our experience of the world is less that of a long life developing through time than that of a network that connects points and intersects with its own skein.' (Foucault 1986: 22). Although it would be difficult, and misleading, to identify a particular date or moment when this occurred, a recognizable *spatial turn* in literary and cultural studies (if not the arts and sciences more generally) has taken place. One cannot help noticing an increasingly spatial or geographic vocabulary in critical texts, with various forms of mapping or cartography being used to survey literary terrains, to plot narrative trajectories, to locate and explore sites, and to project imaginary

coordinates. [...] [T]he spatial or geographical basis of cultural productions have, in recent years, received renewed and forceful critical attentions.

(Tally, 2013, pp. 11–12; author's emphasis)

Robert Tally identifies this '*spatial turn*' as relating to post-war perspectives in the latter half of the twentieth century; 'progress of history in the wake of such destruction, and a changing view of temporal movement may have opened the way to those who demanded that greater attention be paid to spatial concerns.' (Tally, 2013, p. 12) Perspectives on space have developed in some disciplines in this '*spatial turn*'. However, psychoanalytic perspectives on spatial meaning from an unconscious perspective remain relatively underdeveloped theoretically. Harold Searles began to look at human's relationship with the non-human world and the 'matter of regression to a primitive level of thinking, comparable with that found in children and in members of so-called primitive cultures, a level of thinking in which there is a *lack of differentiation between* the concrete and the metaphorical.' (Searles, 1962, p. 23). He also wrote that:

This whole subject may be likened to a vast continent, as yet largely unexplored and uncharted. [...] I am not trying to nail down conclusively, once and for all, this subject of the nonhuman environment in human living but rather to open it up, unprecedently widely and deeply, to the curious, seeking eye.

(Searles, 1987[1960], p. xi)

I consider, that in this book, I am continuing this opening up that Searles writes of, thinking about the non-human environment and the concrete and the metaphorical in relation to the role of the consulting room. In relation to the space of the consulting room, Gary Winship and Shelley MacDonald wrote that:

Containment is both a space and a process that takes place within that space. There has been a growing interest in the intersubjective space or the "analytic third" (Ogden, 2004) of the therapeutic relationship. This is, essentially, the mental amalgam of both client and therapist. [...] We might say that the consulting room itself becomes part of the therapeutic triangulation and operates as the primary container.

(Winship & MacDonald, 2018, p. 73)

Here Winship and MacDonald write of the 'intersubjective space', a space where 'intersubjectivity', between the patient and the therapist takes place. Stern writes of intersubjectivity – that for the infant, 'mental states [...]

become the subject matter of relating. This new sense of a subjective self opens up the possibility for intersubjectivity between infant and parent and operates in a new domain of relatedness.' (Stern, 1985, p. 27). In this book, I am further developing this 'growing interest in the intersubjective space of the therapeutic relationship', which Winship and MacDonald discuss, and I am extending their concept that the consulting room itself 'operates as the 'primary container'. I am suggesting that the consulting room can operate as a 'primary container' and that it can do so as a separate operation from or as a top-up to the containing function of the therapist in the transference. I suggest that the role of the consulting room as a primary container can relate to earlier room use as a primary container (as a replacement or top-up to the mother function), re-spatialised into the consulting room, both as a separate use of the room from the transference, or a top-up to the containing function of the therapist in the transference.

'Spatialisation'

The term 'spatialisation' has been used to describe social meaning related to spaces. Here, I use the term 'spatialisation' not only for the purpose of as-cribing meaning to space, but also to refer to the psychological and physical mechanisms by which this happens, as well as for the motivation behind its use. Rob Shields wrote about 'spatialisation', that it related to: 'approaches to the meaning of the environment which have included work in the area of geography, environmental psychology, and semiotics' (Shields, 1991, p. 11) and he writes that:

> social divisions are spatialised as geographic divisions and how places become 'labelled', much like deviant individuals. Habits such as spatia-lising important conceptual oppositions [...] have been studied as pathologically irrational forms of behaviour [...] Nonetheless it betrays a systematic 'disposition' towards the world (cf. Foucault [...]).
> (Shields, 1991, p. 11)

Shields points to the significance of the meaning that places and spaces give to societal and psychological divisions and concepts. He mentions Foucault, who wrote of spatialisation in political terms, and Shields refers to spatia-lisation as relating to 'pathologically irrational forms of behaviour' and habitual disposition. By comparison, my use of the term spatialisation here is to bring out a different dimension to this phenomenon. I am attempting to bring out the dimension of the meaning, method, and motivation by which these irrational behaviours and dispositions manifest themselves. I propose a formulation and understanding of the concepts of spatialisation that not only takes into account the meaning that is projected onto the environment, but also the psychological and physical mechanisms intrinsic to the process of spatialising whereby this projection takes place. The very idea of an object, including an object of transference, is spatial. That is not about the meaning of spaces, but the creation of meaning through spaces. This differs from the concept of 'psychogeography', which Guy Debord writes of:

> Psychogeography sets for itself the study of the precise laws and specific effects of the geographical environment, whether consciously organised or not, on the emotions and behaviour of the individual [...] to their influence on human feelings, and more generally to any situation or conduct.
>
> (Debord, 2008[1955], p. 23)

Debord suggests that the environment influences the emotions, thoughts, and experiences of the individual in it. I am suggesting that geography (space) not only influences emotions, thoughts, and experiences, but that they are also experienced as spatial through a projection into space and spatialised contents of space, that is, objects. I go on to suggest, that the environment can be 'set up' such as in the Abbey example (see p. 13) to meet the spatialising expectations and needs of the individual and that there is a spatialising interaction of individual and environment. What I argue is that the spatialisation involves a projection of meaning onto – as well as a working of this meaning into the environment. At the primitive level, this is in order to have an experience at all, which is not the same as Debord's influence of space. Therefore, in order to understand more about this, it is important to unfold the motivations for and mechanisms by which such spatialisation is brought about. For the purposes of this thesis, the term spatialisation is used to describe mechanisms that involve a form of projection encompassing physical and psychological aspects. It involves doing things outside the self in the environment, which are physical acts, which only makes sense in a space, that simultaneously involve a psychological projection of meaning. In this study, I am examining spatialisation into rooms and, in particular, the consulting room.

Observation of Phenomena Unaddressed by Current Theories

Here, in thinking about the background and rationale for this book and for the original study shown in Chapter 4, I set out a coherent lodging of my thesis and the relevant precursors on which the thesis is built. In this section, I give examples from historical and cultural data, that show anthropological, and previous clinical and residential care experience. In this section, I show a range of examples of observations of spatialising phenomena demonstrating a range of stages of spatialising from the primitive establishment of objects (pre-transferential), to later re-spatialised transferential stages. These contribute to the formulating of my hypothetical Room-object Spatial Matrix Stages. For example, in the pre-human and early modern human examples, the stone rings inside Bruniquel Cave might be attempts to create a spatialised maternal figure – pre-object, or part-object – a representation of the inside of mother's body, like my hypothesised Room-object Spatial Matrix *Stage 1 – Primal Spatialisation*. Whereas the images of 'Stylized female figures' (Dinnis & Stringer, 2015, p. 136) and 'vulvae' (Dinnis & Stringer, 2015, p. 134) carved into the walls of caves might be more transferential as re-spatialised representation of mother. In the Nigerian village example parts of the environment are spatialised as good and bad part objects, which is also the case in the Westminster Abbey example, and more advanced transferential spatialising occurs in the Chapel of Our Lady of Pew with the actual mother figure a re-projection of the internalised, original, primal spatialisation.

Early Primitive Phenomena in both Modern Humans as Well as Earlier in Neanderthals and Newly Discovered Early Hominins

There is evidence for innate primitive importance of space usage (spatialisation) in both modern humans as well as earlier in the spaces of Neanderthals and a newly discovered earlier hominin. Rob Dinnis and Chris Stringer describe how 40,000 years ago 'caves and rock shelters served as artists' canvases for paintings and engravings. Evocative images range from clearly symbolic, abstract motifs to the stunning naturalistic charcoal depictions.' (Dinnis & Stringer, 2015[2013], pp. 106–107). Other caves are marked out with images of 'Stylized female figures' (Dinnis & Stringer, 2015[2013], p. 136) and 'vulvae' (Dinnis & Stringer, 2015[2013], p. 134) carved into the walls of caves, 'perhaps these figures designated the back of the cave as a sacred place, possibly even a female place; [...] a birthing chamber, safe within the familiarity of the gorge but removed from everyday life.' (Dinnis & Stringer, 2015[2013], p. 135). These examples show that something, perhaps instinct based, is projected and acquires meaning through spatialisation, in which it becomes an object in the first place, which can be introjected and re-projected and therefore captured in a representation.

Stone rings discovered in 2016, inside Bruniquel Cave, (see Fig. 1.1) were 176,000 years old and attributed to Neanderthals. Nadia Drake wrote that '[t]here, several large, layered ring-like structures protruded from the cave floor, the seemingly unmistakable craftwork of builders with a purpose. [...] The mysterious structures are built from nearly 400 stalagmites' (Drake, 2016, pp. 2–3). They are 'craftwork' with a meaning and a purpose. Stringer writes, 'these must have been made by early Neanderthals, the only known inhabitants of Europe at this time. [...]' If there is still – buried debris from occupation, it would help us to determine whether this was [...] something which had more symbolic or ritual significance.' (Stringer, 2016, p. 1)

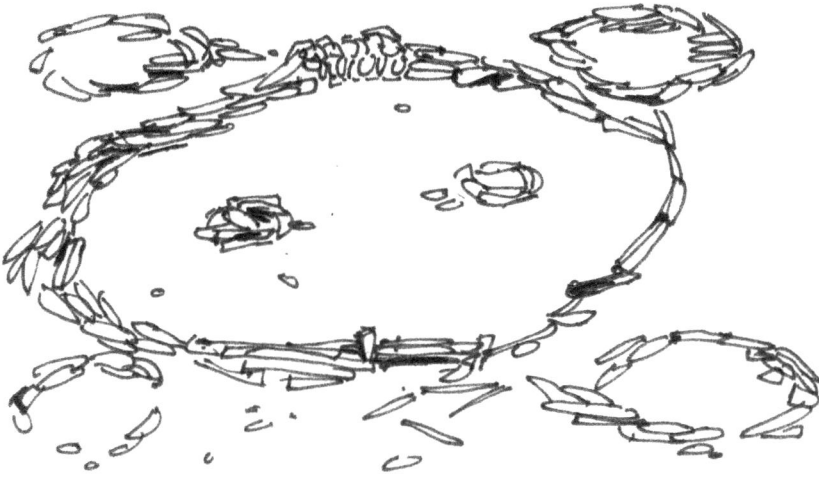

Figure 1.1 Structures in the Bruniquel cave. Drawing by D. Wright.

Stringer is identifying the age and significance of the find as being unique as a Neanderthal-built structure of that age, as well as considering the usage of the rings as being made for ritual purposes. This is the earliest example of a crafted, meaning-made space that might be attempting to create a spatialised maternal figure, like my hypothetical Room-object Spatialisation Matrix Stage 1 – *Primal Spatialisation*. Ninian Smart wrote:

> There is ample evidence that religious rites were practised in early prehistoric times and it may well be that the sense of the sacred has been part of man's experience from the beginning. It is notable that before the emergence of the human species proper (*homo sapiens*), Neanderthal Man – some 150,000 years ago – practised the ritual interment of the dead. This seems to point to a belief in an afterlife of some kind and to belief in an 'invisible' world.
>
> (Smart, 1971[1969], p. 33)

Lee Berger and his team published their findings in September 2015 of bones in the Dinaledi chamber of the Rising Star Caves in South Africa (Fig. 1.2 shows a cross-section on the far right on the diagram) of an earlier hominin (Homa naledi) than Neanderthals practicing ritual burial in the cave space. As Berger et al discuss; 'Based on current evidence, our preferred explanation for the accumulation of Homo naledi fossils in the Dinaledi Chamber is deliberate body disposal [...]. Our interpretation of events raises questions about the meaning of deliberate and repeated body disposal to this ancient

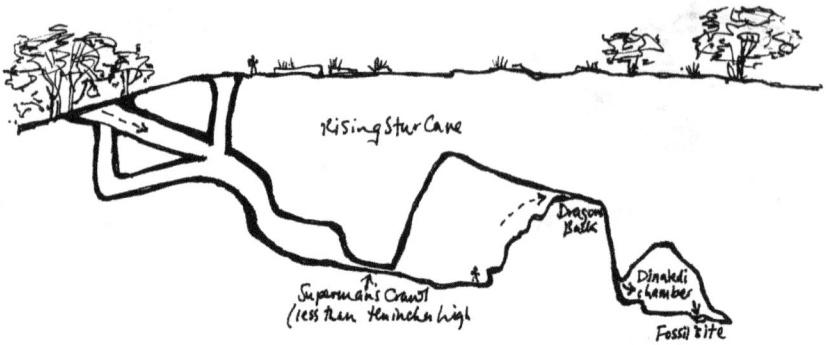

Figure 1.2 The Rising Star cave. Drawing by D. Wright.

group of individuals' and that Homo naledi might have had 'distinctive patterns of behavioural complexity' (Berger et al., 2015, pp. 5–6).

So here we have evidence of newly discovered pre-humans apparently also showing signs of the use and meaning making of space, place, and objects. Jamie Shreeve wrote in his commentary on Berger and his team's paper: 'Until now only *Homo sapiens,* and possibly some archaic humans such as the Neanderthals, are known to have treated their dead in such a ritualised manner. [...] The notion of such a small-brained creature exhibiting such complex behaviour seems so unlikely that many other researchers have simply refused to credit it.' (Shreeve, 2015, p. 53). All of these examples show, what I am suggesting is a primitive human (and pre-human) mechanism of spatialising where meaning (individually or collectively) was created through the spatialisation. In relation to Smart's thoughts above, about an 'afterlife [...] in an 'invisible' world' (Smart, 1971[1969], p. 33), perhaps this, in a primitive sense, means life in another place, which is a form of spatialisation. This may perhaps relate this world post-life to the pre-life womb space (also an 'invisible' world) so it is a pre-object spatialisation, post-object; a post-object spatialisation. The Rising Star Caves here, and the Reliquary (see p. 14&15) show aspects of this womb-like space with the idea of an entrance but an impossible exit for the bones as they sit permanently in the womb-like area. This will be discussed further in Chapter 8, as I suggest that this can be thought of as an *End Room-object* space.

Observation of Phenomena in Nigerian Village Setting

The next example is of a village in the Oban hills area of Nigeria, where I worked in the early 1990s, and observed the dividing up of spaces into sacred and profane as a way of managing the environment and living within it. This is what I am calling spatialising – the village itself is spatial and is moved around and in and out of using spatial ritual. The village was surrounded by rainforest that was considered dangerous and threatening, containing wild animals, reptiles, and insects. Since, here, the outside of the village was dangerous, 'bad' and the inside safe, 'good' (see Klein (1946) in Chapter 3, p. 64), outside dangers, as well as inside social cohesion, were managed by a variety of spatialising techniques. These included rituals performed by the chief and the elders in the central meeting-building and the elders in the elders' meeting area (the highest point in the village), as well as rituals at the sacred tree which spanned the nearby river. The community believes that, in order to safely move in and out of the village, all members of the village transform into animals. The outside of the village is the profane/bad/dangerous area and the inside is sacred/good and safe. Within the array of the village are the designated sacred locations – the sacred tree above the river, the highest point, and the meeting building. These locations and the rituals that take place there manage the sacred and profane by keeping safety and danger in place. As E. Bolaji Idowu writes; 'The sages of the Yoruba have always admitted that there are certain apparatus or aspects of religion that were originally no more than interventions of priestcraft either for the purpose of serving political or civic ends for the 'good' of the community' (Idowu, 1973, p. 35), however, he goes on to say that 'with reference to the religion of Southern Nigeria [...] the fact about the use of material emblems is that to Africans, the material has no meaning apart from the spiritual; it is the spiritual that informs the material and gives it whatever quality and meaning it has. The material, therefore, can only be, at best, technically a symbol.' (Idowu, 1973, p. 125). What Idowu is describing is a spatialisation of the environment creating meaning for functioning.

Mircea Eliade (1959), wrote that the 'sacred tree, the sacred stone are not adored as stone or tree; they are worshipped precisely because they are *hierophanies*, because they show something that is no longer stone or tree but the *sacred*' (Eliade, 1959, p. 12). The meaning of the array of the space and the objects within it are changed – changed and manipulated – in order to create a required meaning by psychological projection and physical manipulation. Karl Figlio writes of: 'a culture steeped in animism and magic, in which people believe they make things happen through the power of words or other acts. But in animistic culture, words or acts imitate or invoke what appears to the senses.' (Figlio, 2000, p. 12). I understand these processes as acts of spatialising, including ritual belief, projecting, and physical manipulation performed to control instincts or a nascent internal world. Eliade wrote:

> One of the outstanding characteristics of traditional societies is the opposition that they assume between their inhabited territory and the

unknown and indeterminable space that surrounds it. [...] At first sight this cleavage in space appears to be due to the opposition between an inhabited and organized – hence cosmicized – territory and the unknown space that extends beyond its frontiers; on one side there is a cosmos, on the other a chaos. [...] The sacred reveals absolute reality and at the same time makes orientation possible; hence it *founds the world* in the sense that it fixes the limits and establishes the order of the world.

(Eliade 1959, pp. 29–30)

The sacred in Eliade's conception thus ties in with and is constitutive of the ordered world; it defines and fixes its limits. What Eliade has described as 'chaos' is separate from what is good and sacred inside. Harold Searles writes that in pre-modern societies people were:

at the mercy of an animistic, and often anthropomorphised, nonhuman environment which was basically hostile, chaotic, utterly uncontrollable. It may perhaps be counted man's proudest achievement that he has come, largely through the medium of scientific endeavour, to realise so many of his uniquely human potentialities, to free himself to the extent that he has from an ancient, overwhelming awe of the nonhuman.

(Searles, 1987[1960], p. 7)

but goes on to point out that 'science itself, which along with the more ascetic components of the Christian religion has tended to foster in man a conviction that he is basically alien to his nonhuman environment, has yielded abundantly convincing data, from various sources, to show him how closely akin he is to that environment.' (Searles, 1987[1960], p. 8). Searles is saying that science may allow for rationalisation about the 'chaotic', which Eliade writes of, but that we are still 'closely akin' to the environment. I am suggesting that spatialising, even if with more individually based projections than larger group ones that I write of in the Nigeria example, or a large-scale system of space organising such as the Chinese Feng Shui one, designed for spatialising purposes, to control and organise spaces with projected instinctual feeling (such as fear or anxiety) safely organised, is still a basic and primitive mechanism for functioning. As Karl Figlio writes; 'Harold Searles argues that the pull of identification reaches beyond primitive object relations, even beyond the non-human world, and reaches right back to the inanimate world' (Figlio, 2000, p. 11). I argue that there is a primitive human mechanism to spatialise involving projection and actual physical manipulation of physical spaces in order to control psychological space.

Observation of Phenomena in Westminster Abbey

Along similar lines, Karl Figlio and Barry Richards (2003) write that 'containment':

> occurred in premodern societies, but, in the absence of continuous physical reminders of the social, it would have been carried more by the intense, if episodic, regimes of psychic management of rituals and by manifest symbolic associations, as in the layout of a cathedral.
>
> (Figlio & Richards, 2003, p. 412)

Figlio and Richards refer in this context to the 'shared illusion' (Figlio & Richards, 2003, p. 420) of society 'generated through collective imagination' (Figlio & Richards, 2003, p. 420). In Westminster Abbey, as with any religious building for any culture or period, the building is designed and shaped in a way that is required of the function and meaning of the space. As Jacques Le Goff wrote; 'Indo-European tradition had evolved a way of interpreting space symbolically' (Le Goff, 1992[1985], p. 85). The 'Art' of creating a space of spatialised cultural meaning in this way is described by Frances Yates: 'This art seeks to memorize through a technique of impressing 'places' and 'images' on memory […] an art which uses contemporary architecture for its memory places and contemporary imagery for its images.' (Yates, 1966, p. 11).

Pilgrims passing through the space of the abbey journeyed through an experience that was psychological, emotional, and physical with many different spaces marked out with art works containing symbols giving context to and providing an authoritative understanding of the experience of the individual. Johan Huizinga writes that '[t]he spirit of the Middle Ages, still plastic and naïve longs to give concrete shape to every conception. Every thought seeks expression in an image […] [b]y this tendency to embodiment in visible forms all holy concepts' (Huizinga, (1990[1924]), p. 147). This representation, albeit concrete, is not the same, as the primitive stone rings in the Bruniquel Cave. It may be retrogressive, but it is not the same as object creating. This representation, as with the cave paintings, is the more advanced introjected and projected spatialising (as with my hypothesised Room-object Spatial Matrix, *Stage 2, Room-object*). The individuals' projections, associations, and unconscious fantasies connected to or prompted by that space, are thus facilitated, reinforced – and also: limited – by the construction of the space in the architecture and art works and relate to the 'common symbolism' (Freud, 1961[1923], p. 242) contained in these.

There are dense layers of meaning here; there is the space created with signs and symbols to facilitate the needs and expectations of the pilgrim and to provide a facilitating setting for a re-creation of an experience. There is then the facilitation of the emotions connected with the meaning. In order to do this, the separated spaces are in a relationship with each other, they are divided up with different meanings as part of the overall control of meaning and experience. This dividing up of space can involve, as shown in the example of the village, clearly defined areas of good or bad, safety or danger, sacred or profane, regarding the spatial structures within which ideas find their expression, as well as the margins of such structures. Mary Douglas (1966) writes that

> all margins are dangerous. If they are pulled this way or that the shape of fundamental experience is altered. Any structure of ideas is vulnerable at its margins. We should expect the orifices of the body to symbolise its specially vulnerable points. Matter issuing from them is marginal stuff of the most obvious kind its spittle, blood, milk, urine, faeces or tears by simply issuing forth have traversed the boundary of the body.
>
> (Douglas (1999 [1966]), p. 122)

Margins, according to Douglas, can be dangerous because they are borders between domains that, psychically, need to be protected from confusion for psychic stability. Here, Douglas is in tune with psychoanalytic thinking about what Donald Meltzer calls 'zonal confusion' (Meltzer, 2019[1974], p. 113). As can be seen in the Nigerian village example, the sacred location keeps the profane location in position. The meaning of the sacred location holds the profane at bay and the proximity of the profane throws the meaning of the sacred location into relief. In the case of Westminster Abbey, the building's inside and outside also represent the limits of the sacred and profane respectively. As with the village model, spatialisation is employed to keep these locations separate and protect the sacred from the profane. Gargoyles were created to cast the bad off the building into the outside like tears or sweat out of a body, purifying and keeping sacred the contents inside. If we take the 'body' of the Abbey to represent the human body, Douglas's observation that 'body symbolism is part of the common stock of symbols, deeply emotive because of the individual's experience' (Douglas, 1999[1966]), p. 122) can be brought to bear on the building. The insides of the Abbey can thus be seen to represent the original object of spatialisation – the mother's body, the most powerful and potent object of spatialisation. The nave and the aisles (see Fig. 1.3), like the main arteries of the body, pass through different locations of particular sacred meaning (such as chapels) towards the most sacred area behind the screen; the reliquary (see Fig. 1.4). The reliquary (The Shrine of Saint Edward the Confessor) is like the womb of the building where the most sacred and powerful objects in the Abbey, the relics, are contained. The sacred bones contain the greatest most efficacious good projection and relate to a fantasy of merging with the

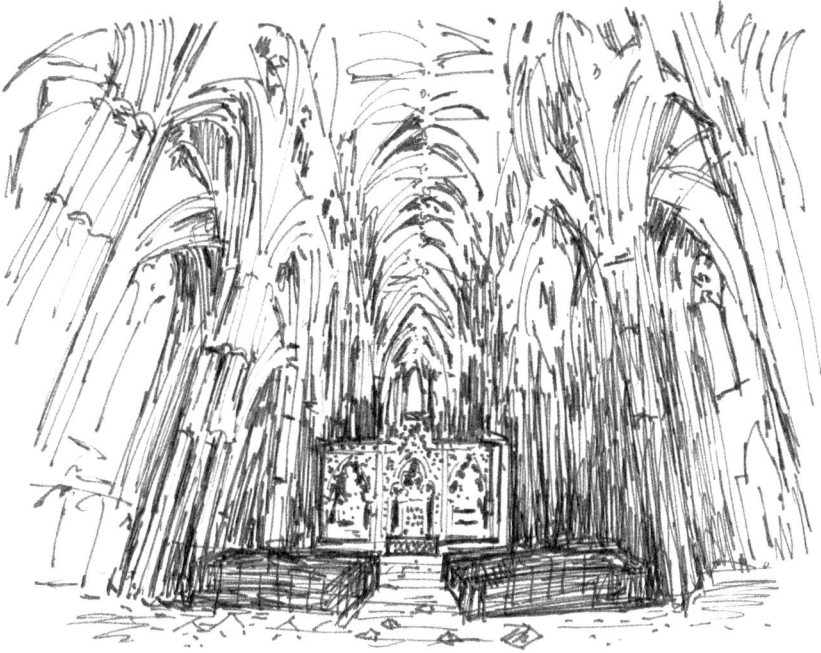

Figure 1.3 Drawing of the nave of Westminster Abbey. Drawing by D. Wright.

sacred bones providing 'comfort and salvation' (Miccoli, 1990[1987], p. 47). In the reliquary, the arched kneeling spaces (see the 3 along the bottom of Fig. 1.4) afford the pilgrim an opportunity to get even closer in to the sacred relics, the treasure. However, as with the womb, it can be approached but never quite reached, creating a constant seeking to control that experience and that space. As Figlio writes 'I have argued that we are driven to know mother from the outside and the inside' (Figlio, 2000, p. 21). As with the village model, there is dividing up of the sacred space inside into various localised areas (chapels) of sacred which keep profane in position outside. The Chapel of Our Lady of Pew (see Figs. 1.5 and 1.6), 'Pew' meaning a small chapel or enclosure, venerates Mary, Mother of Jesus, and contains a pink alabaster statue of Mary holding the baby Jesus. According to the Dean and Chapter of Westminster Abbey:

> The painted vaulting of this recess with its carved boss of the Assumption [see Fig. 1.5] dates from the second half of the fourteenth century and in the back wall of the recess, facing the Ambulatory, was a shallow niche with a bracket on which stood an image of our

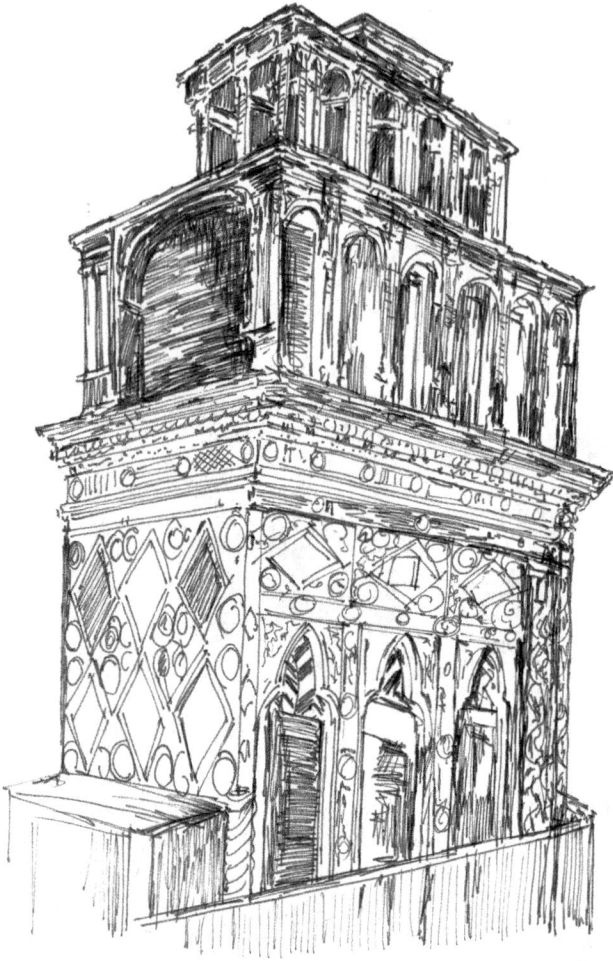

Figure 1.4 Drawing of the shrine of Edward the Confessor. Drawing by D. Wright.

Lady [...] The walls of the recess were elaborately painted and are studded with hooks evidently for votive offering. The outer doorway with its painted wooden half-gates and iron bracket for an alms-box are also original.

(Dean & Chapter of Westminster, 1994 [1988], p. 59)

For the pilgrim, this chapel was a spatialising experience. At the womb-like entrance, the pilgrim would deposit money in the alms box for the poor, so they might projectively be looked after in the way in which the pilgrim hopes to be looked after by the mother, defending against the

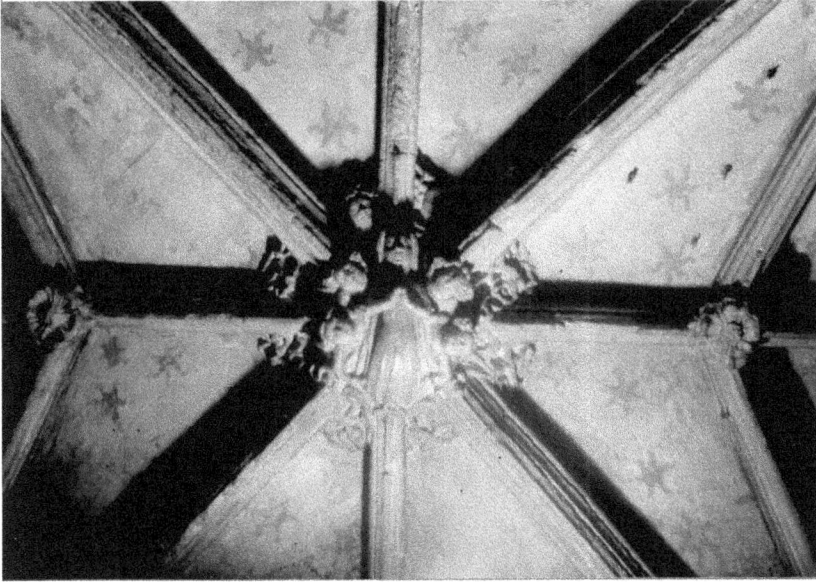

Figure 1.5 The Chapel of Our Lady of Pew ceiling, in Westminster Abbey. Photograph by D. Wright.

possibility of the mother function not being good enough. The small dark chapel which glows pink, creating a womb-like interior, (see Fig. 1.6) allowed the pilgrim to get close in towards mother, whilst above them the ribbed ceiling encloses them, with additional mother imagery on the central boss (see Fig. 1.5). Around the statue of the mother there are hooks on which to hang 'votive offerings', objects to gain favour from the transferential mother figure. This is a more advanced spatialising stage of a re-projection of the internalised, original spatialisation of mother into an actual transferential object mother figure, like the therapist, to spatialise into (as in my hypothesised Room-object Spatial Matrix *Stage 4 – Consulting Room-object + Transference*).

A more recent example of spatialising, into the domestic space of rooms, is given by Judith Flanders who writes:

> In the 1960s, builders renovating a house in north London found, bricked up behind a fireplace, a basket holding two shoes, a candlestick and a drinking vessel […]: votive offerings to the house-gods of the 16th Century, resurfacing in the twentieth. Houses, according to myth, folk tale and legend, have souls, and possibly even minds. While we may no longer subscribe to these beliefs on a conscious level, many small rituals based on those beliefs were performed until recently: clocks were

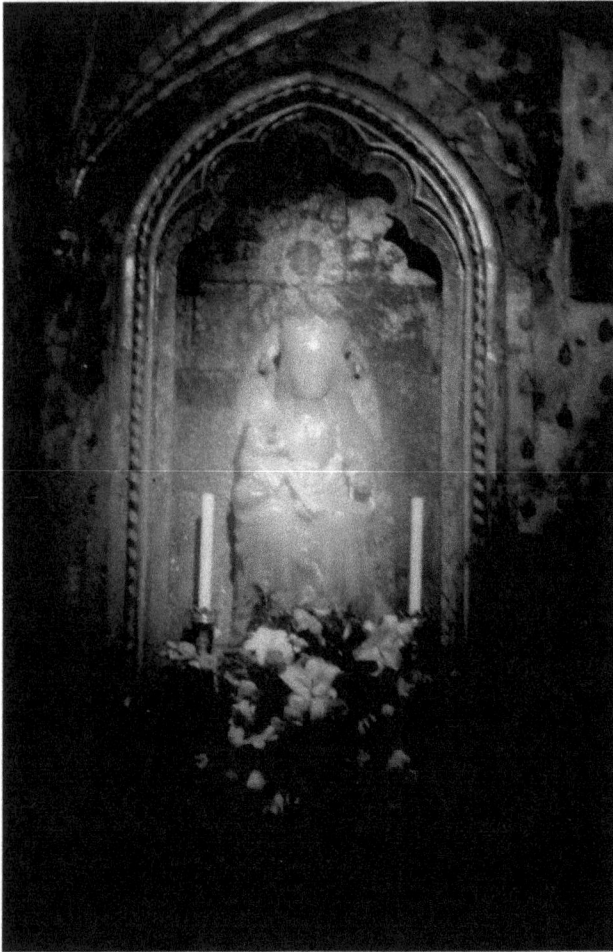

Figure 1.6 The Chapel of Our Lady of Pew interior, in Westminster Abbey. Photograph by D. Wright.

stopped and mirrors veiled on the death of a member of the household, while on the day of a funeral window – blinds were habitually drawn, covering the house's 'eyes'.

(Flanders, 2014, p. 165)

I suggest that this can be thought of as a spatialising projection of aspects of protective family members into the actual walls of a room, these objects are already humanised, already introjected from a spatialised, maternal transference. As well as this the house itself is anthropomorphised, with its own 'eyes' (to see outside danger) and 'mind' that can contain and protect the inhabitants inside.

Observation of Phenomena in Residential Care

I observed phenomena relating to client's relationships with rooms, when I worked as a residential care manager in a home for people with mild learning difficulties and mental health problems, before and during my psychotherapy training. I was used to working with resident's spatialising and manipulating of physical space to control the psychological space. This included ritualising before going out of the building or out of their bedrooms, much like the ritualising and spatialising in the Nigerian village scenario. I repeatedly observed the importance of the client's bedrooms to them. An example of this can be seen in the case of one of the residential clients, Mr X who has frequent psychotic episodes and went through long periods of not wanting to leave his bedroom. It was the only place where it seemed that he felt he had some sort of mind. He occasionally went to the kitchen where he colonised one end with his music system and where playing CD's was a form of control of the environment. Another control was refusing food and only drinking milk, like an infant. Mr X had a mentally ill mother and violent Father with whom, as a child, there were a lot of experiences with guns. It seemed that his room was not only the safest place but provided the safest feedback.

Observation of Phenomena in the Physical Space of the Psychotherapy Room

Whilst working as a psychotherapist, I have observed phenomena relating to patient's relationship with the consulting room, which at times seems unrelated to the transference to me. It appears to be a very specific relationship with the room, much like the example of Mr X above, that fulfils a function for the patient as separate from me. This includes patients' ritualistic behaviours whilst moving in and out of the consulting room, using the toilet, hallways, and interim areas, including the use of door and objects such as cushions, all of which I have observed to be heightened during consulting room moves. I have also noticed that room moves bring out the meaning of patient's relationships with the consulting room as well as rooms from their past. While the current view is that unconscious communications of the patient relate to either transference, or an avoidance of the transference, I think it is important to recognise the more primitive, pre-transferential states of mind. I am also suggesting that it is a place where patient may go that relates to their relationship with rooms which they originally formed as a top-up to the mother function or at times replacement of that and that this is an important communication to understand.

Clinical Example of Spatialising in the Consulting Room; Mr A

An example of this can be seen in clinical work with a patient, Mr A, mid-30s, who's presenting problems were the impact that meeting strangers for sex from on-line forums was having on him and his long-term relationship, as well as a residual difficulty around weight and eating that, although not the reason for beginning the work, was an ongoing difficulty. He had spent a lot of time thinking about and working on his weight, having been very overweight as a teen and in his early 20s, he had since successfully done a number of diets to control this. Mr A is an intelligent and erudite man with a successful career in computer engineering. He liked thinking about the difficulties he brought by factually picking them apart like parts of a machine, ordering them, and trying to understand how they work (much like his approach to his job as an engineer). His dreams often involved computing conundrums and tasks from his work or personal pursuit that he endlessly fixed and worked out. He disliked talking about his mother and father, particularly his mother – this felt 'off limits'. His mother left his father, taking him and his brother, when he was 7, after she had an affair. They lived in a series of different houses throughout the rest of his childhood, some work related (hotels) and some rented. So, he had a number of early rooms and bedrooms and was also responsible at an early age for looking after their home environment including cooking whilst his Mother worked long shifts. In a session, about a year after beginning working with me;

On arrival in the consulting room, Mr A turned round and banged into the large Victorian mirror on top of a side-board unit which he had never noticed before as it was behind him. He was immediately fascinated with it and he touched it, patted it and gazed at it. He said that the dark wood of it and the shape reminded him of an enormous dark wooden dresser which was in his first home living/dining room as a child.

Mr A said "I must have been very small- I can't remember – it was always there- I remember reaching up to open the drawers. It must have been very tall."

He said several times it must have been very tall whist touching the wood on the frame and looking up and down the mirror and the shelf parts to it. He then said, "Inside the drawers were family games and place mats for the table."

He thought for a while whilst looking at the mirror and touching the wood on the frame, and then said it was reminiscent, as an item, of order and calm, and when his parents were still together. He said that when his Mother left his Father with his brother and him, they took the dresser with them (and it was the only piece of furniture that they took from the house), and that at first it was very meaningful to him as a reminder of his home and then, as time went on, and they had lived in many different houses since leaving the original family home he had lived with his Mother and Father, he feels that it became less and less meaningful. He said that could not remember what happened to it in the end. He became very sad when he thought this.

This object in the consulting, the mirror and sideboard, became imbued with the meaning of the original dresser in the original family home room which felt "ordered and calm" like when his mother and father were still together, therefore Oedipally more ordered than after when he had to look after things for mother including the home, and before the disordered move from the family home and living in different spaces. It was a safe room in a safe house before living in many. The mirror and sideboard felt, at that moment of recognition and sensory memory of the colour of the wood, the carving and the feel of the wood and so on, spontaneously created a range of spatialised emotions, thoughts, and perceptions. Mr A's relationships with the sideboard in the consulting room became intense and important in a re-imagining and experiencing this feeling of early primitive mother and father space, his original room space. This created an emotional engagement with the work that touched on primitive and unconscious material and feelings that were important in the work, in representing both a happy and calm time of order and the deep sadness of its loss. Gazing at and stroking the sideboard was like the safe object mother where father is there too, to keep order with Mother, and the safe Room-object space, where the sideboard keeps the order of the family activities (games) and eating (placemats), all of which was lost when the separation with Father and the house occurred. This enabled a safer engagement in the consulting room, with emotions about that early space, and it became important in understanding the unsafe and un-ordered sexual and eating behaviour and the feelings around this.

We can see spatialising again, in a session from the following year of work with Mr A, when he discussed on several occasions on arrival to the Consulting room, for several weeks, that there were residual bits of Christmas decoration tinsel remaining stuck to my door knocker with sticky tape, where I had removed the Christmas wreath that had been made from tinsel without removing all the sticky tape. On first mentioning it, Mr A said that he had felt like taking the sticky tape off himself, it was "so tempting to do it". My countertransference was that I felt guilty that it had been a cheap wreath that I had carelessly taken down and that my housekeeping was remiss, and my immediate reaction was to think I must remove that. However, I kept forgetting and my guilt in the counter-transference stopped it getting thought about properly:

Eventually, after several weeks, Mr A pulled a bit of the tinselly sticky tape off the knocker himself, and brought it in with him to the consulting room. I experienced my guilt as compounded by my initial lack of care for the space, day in day out continuing to forget, and then him doing the house keeping for me - this was Mother in the transference, but more than that, during the session, Mr A was criticising himself for how long it has been that he has been planning to make his eating more ordered since the last diet;

He said, "I actually finished in October, have I been talking about it for that long?"

I said, "that's very critical of yourself, maybe criticising yourself is easier than other people"

He said, "Oh, I have been criticising someone at work. He left a lot of work for me to do when I came back after Easter, he never does anything properly". I then linked this to the Christmas decoration and the feeling of him having to look after everything, including the consulting room and entrance to it.

His spatialised behaviour around the door knocker – as the boundary of the house, related to his experiences as me leaving it messy, and therefore something felt disordered (a *Stage 2 'Room- object'* experience) and it was an uncontained entrance to the space, as the house in a primitive way felt disordered. This is not only a transferential experience where I was the mother, who disorders things and who he has to clean up after but also he has to contain the space. But it is also a re-spatialised experience of the early 'Room-object' spaces that began with 'order', (with the spatialised early 'Primal Spatialisation' experience of the mirror/dresser which we could think of as the 'ordered' pre-separated 'Room-object' when the family system felt ordered. But these early room spaces became slowly less and less ordered, the meaning of the dresser further away and this disordered room space that has to be cleaned and ordered was re-experienced here.

Some patients take a long time to engage with me as a therapist but have an important attachment to the consulting room that can keep the therapy work going for weeks or even years until they can begin to relate to the idea of me being in the room as well. Not only that, but their relationship with the spatial array of rooms, building and streets around the consulting room can also be of great importance. What I suggest is that the room space and its contents can play a large part in the therapeutic process at a largely unconscious and very primitive level and remains a place to retreat into, providing a safe haven as a deflection from the transference when it becomes intense. I am opening up an area rarely spoken about, in a literature that sees the objects and the space of the consulting room solely as aspects of the analyst: as the analyst's consulting room or as features of the analyst displayed in the consulting room. I will be providing more detailed clinical examples in Chapters 4, 5, and 6 with some further examples in Chapter 8.

Observation of Phenomena in the Virtual Space of the Psychotherapy Room

During the course of 2020 events relating to the Covid-19 virus pandemic, led to the practice of psychotherapy changing in a very spatial and potentially long-lasting way – with remote, phone, and online virtual working the norm since lockdown. In Chapter 6, I will show a range of clinical examples of patients who have and have not been working in a physical room and their spatial usage and spatialising into the virtual space of the consulting room and ways in which this can be thought about.

For Mr A, after moving to the 'Virtual consulting room' his normal dreams involving ordering things that he is working on at work, changed to a dream about houses that he has lived in. In one disordered scene; a flatmate is forced to inject a drug, in another scene and room a flatmate is being sick over a sink and there is no wall so it goes down the outside of the room. These are broken up and disordered rooms, partly relating to the damaged Room-objects as well as concerns about family in relation to Covid where things also feel broken up. Like many patients, Mr A explored the possibilities, in different ways, of the use of video calls for having sessions in the Virtual consulting room. Examples of this in relation to other patients' experiences will be discussed in detail in Chapter 6, this included the opportunity to show me the room or rooms that they are in and think about spatialising aspects of these or activities in them or objects in them, that get shown and demonstrated, such as, in the case of Mr A, a mixing deck that he bought and how to use it and what it means to him. This also included the 'screen share' mechanism on video calls that enable the patient to show images to me in more detail that if they brought them to the room. Jordan Bate and Norka Malberg (2020) wrote in 'Containing the Anxieties of Children, Parents, and Families from a Distance During the Coronavirus Pandemic' about the adaptation by the therapist to the virtual online consulting room where a child patient uses 'screen share' in the play, to create another dimension to the work. First, the child dressed in their Father's nurse uniform and talk about his fighting the 'corona monster' he then shows a video clip on 'screen share' about a kangaroo that wants to drive a truck and all the catastrophic things that can happen. The therapist reports that; 'Though I am uncertain that my patient can work at this symbolic level and aware that we are miles apart, so I cannot offer the usual ways of containment (sandbox, sensory toys, or simply my physical presence), I nevertheless continue.' (Bate & Malberg, 2020). The therapist gave an interpretation relating the Kangaroo's potential disasters to the 'corona monster' presenting danger and they are like the Kangaroo – this inter-pretation was well accepted and enables a reflection that Dad fights the monster. So, Bate and Malberg are able to demonstrate the efficacy of the use of 'screen share' and flexibility and receptiveness to patient's different spatial activity in the Virtual consulting room and its meaning.

Yonit Shulman and Abraham Saroff likewise, in their paper, '"Imagination for Two" Child Psychotherapy during Coronavirus Outbreak: Building a Space for Play When Space Collapses', also discuss the 'screen share' feature showing the creative possibility of it, that adds significantly to the work generally as a contribution to the Virtual consulting room space and possible therapeutic process therein that I explore extensively in Chapter 6. They write that the patient 'used the "share screen" feature of the Zoom application in order to show me photos of herself as a baby, tacitly sharing with me more of her early history and the losses she suffered since, issues we could rarely dis-cuss openly before' (Shulman and Saroff, 2020, p. 343).

In the case of Mr A, after the death of his Grandfather, from Covid-related illness, (not long after the death of his grandmother, also related to Covid) he discussed the funeral and memories of his Grandfather in a ses-sion. He showed me photographs on 'screen share' of his grandfather (and some of him as a child with his Grandfather), that he was given by family members around the time of the funeral. He talked about his grandfather, his relationship with his grandfather, and during this screen sharing he suddenly came across a photograph of his early living/dining room from his early family home with the large wooden dresser (as discussed earlier, in relation to the sideboard in the consulting room) in it, which felt like a surprise for him and very important. He talked about the dresser again, what was on the shelves and drawers, about the wood, and there was thinking about the loss of that room (and order of it and the contents of the drawers and how calm it was), the dresser, grandfather and the consulting room and sideboard/mirror there. Mr A then did a spontaneous online search to see if he could find a photograph of his grandparents' house from when he was young, that they had sold more recently to move to a bungalow that was 'meaningless' to him. He wanted to show me their meaningful house. Then he unexpectedly found a house spec from when the house had sold years ago with lots of photographs with it, showing all of the original furniture and items from when he was young. This was extremely emotional and shocking for him, and he unexpectedly found it, rather like the scene in the consulting room when he touched the mirror, that this stimulated the primitive spatialised memories of the dresser. Here the 'screen share' ex-perience of looking at these pictures of their house, as they had lived in it, in which all the familiar things were, and me looking at it with him, was very meaningful, as he reflected that his grandparents' house had been a safe, ordered and constant after his parents split up and he lived in many different houses and rooms. 'Screen share' has been an important visual and spatial sharing for Mr A, including the plans for the major house renovation that he is creating with his partner, including a "specially designed office", a creation of a 'Room-object' outside the consulting room.

This chapter introduces the background and rationale for thinking about and conceptualising the observed phenomena of transference to the consulting room space which can be thought of as being both separate, as well as related to the transference to the therapist. This begins with proposed use of the words 'spatialisation' and shows examples from historical and anthropological spatialisation from; palaeontological use of space; examples from Nigeria and Westminster Abbey; the Residential Care setting as well as clinical, which contribute to a foundation alongside psychoanalytic spatial concepts as well as an analysis of Sigmund Freud's Consulting room in Chapter 2, on which to build a new conceptual formulation that considers spatialisation developmentally, the Room-object Spatial Matrix, in Chapter 3.

Figure References

Figure 1.1: Structures in the Bruniquel Cave. Drawing by D. Wright, sketched from illustration 'A 3D reconstruction of the structures in Bruniquel Cave, 'Rendering by Xavier Muth/Get in Situ/Archeotransfer/Archeovision-SHS-3D; Base Photographique Pascal Mora' in Drake, N. (2016) Neanderthals Built Mysterious Stone Circles. [online][Accessed 12 September 2016]. Available from: http://news.national geographic.com/2016/05/Neanderthals-caves-rings-building-francerchaeology/.

Figure 1.2: The Rising Star Cave. Drawing by D. Wright, sketched from illustration (Page 38) in Shreeve, J. (2015) 'Mystery Man'. National Geographic. Volume 228. Number 4: 30–57).

Figure 1.3: Drawing of the Nave of Westminster Abbey. Drawing by D. Wright. *Reproduced with permission of Palgrave Macmillan from* Wright, D. (2019) *'Spatialisation and the Fomenting of Political Violence' in Fomenting Political Violence – Fantasy, Language, Media, Action.' (pp. 167–187), Eds. Steffen Kruger, Karl Figlio, Barry Richards. Switzerland, Palgrave Macmillan. Reproduced with permission of Palgrave Macmillan.*

Figure 1.4: Drawing of The Shrine of Saint Edward the Confessor. Drawing by D. Wright. *Reproduced with permission of Palgrave Macmillan from* Wright, D. (2019) *'Spatialisation and the Fomenting of Political Violence' in Fomenting Political Violence – Fantasy, Language, Media, Action.' (pp. 167–187), Eds. Steffen Kruger, Karl Figlio, Barry Richards. Switzerland, Palgrave Macmillan. Reproduced with permission of Palgrave Macmillan.*

Figure 1.5: The Chapel of Our Lady of Pew ceiling, in Westminster Abbey. Photograph by D. Wright.

Figure 1.6: The Chapel of Our Lady of Pew interior, in Westminster Abbey. Photograph by D. Wright.

References

Bate J., and Malberg, N. (2020) Containing the Anxieties of Children, Parents and Families from a Distance During the Coronavirus Pandemic. *Journal of Contemporary Psychotherapy.* 50: 285–294. Published online: 14 July 2020, 10.1007/s10879-020-09466-4 © Springer Science+Business Media, LLC, part of Springer Nature 2020.

Berger L. R. et al. http://elifesciences.org/content/4/e09561 04/10/2015 Geological and taphonomic context for the new hominin species Homo naledi from the Dinaledi Chamber, South Africa – See more at: http://elifesciences.org/content/4/e09561#.dpuf Paul HGM Dirks, Lee R Berger, Eric M Roberts, Jan D Kramers, John Hawks, Patrick S Randolph-Quinney, Marina Elliott, Charles M Musiba, Steven E Churchill, Darryl J de Ruiter, Peter Schmid, Lucinda R Backwell, Georgy A Belyanin, Pedro Boshoff, K Lindsay Hunter, Elen M Feuerriegel, Alia Gurtov, James du G Harrison, Rick Hunter, Ashley Kruger, Hannah Morris, Tebogo V Makhubela, Becca Peixotto, Steven Tucker - See more at: http://elifesciences.org/content/4/e09561#.dpuf

Dean & Chapter of Westminster, (1994 [1998]) *Westminster Abbey Official Guide.* Norwich: Jarrold Publishing.

Debord, G. (2008 [1955]) Introduction to a Critique of Urban Geography (1955). Tr. Ken Knabb *Critical Geographies A Collection of Readings* (2008) Eds. Harald Bauder & Salvatore Engel–Di Mauro. Edition, http://www.praxis-epress.org/availablebooks/introcriticalgeog.html, Kelowna, British Columbia, Canada. Praxis (e) Press, http://wwwpraxix-epress.org

Dinnis, R. and Stringer, C. (2015 [2013]) *Britain – One Million Years of the Human Story.* London: Natural History Museum.

Douglas, M. (1999 [1966]) *Purity and Danger An analysis of the concepts of pollution and taboo.* London: Routledge.

Drake, N. (2016) Neanderthals Built Mysterious Stone Circles. [online]. [Accessed 12September2016]. Available from: http://news.national geographic.com/2016/05/Neanderthals-caves-rings-building-france-archaeology/

Eliade, M. (1959) *The Sacred and the Profane the Nature of Religion.* (Trans. Trask, W.R.). New York and London: Harcourt Brace & Jovanovich.

Figlio, K. (2000) *Psychoanalysis, Science and Masculinity.* London and Philadelphia: Whurr Publishers.

Figlio, K., Richards, B. (2003) The Containing Matrix of the Social. American Imago, 60:407–428.

Flanders, J. (2014) *The Making of Home.* London: Atlantic Books.

Foucault, M. (1986) Of Other Spaces. trans. Jay Miskowiec, *Diacritics 16 (spring)* 22–27.

Freud, S. (1957 [1915]) Instincts and their Vicissitudes. Tr. & ed. James Strachey *et al. Standard Edition of the Complete Psychological Works of Sigmund Freud*, vol XIV. London: Hogarth Press and the Institute of Psychoanalysis. 109–140.

Freud, S. (1961 [1923]). The Ego and the Id. Tr. & ed. James Strachey *et al. Standard Edition of the Complete Psychological Works of Sigmund Freud*, vol XIX. London: Hogarth Press and the Institute of Psychoanalysis.1–66.

Huizinga, J. (1990 [1924]) *The Waning of the Middle Ages.* London: Penguin.

Idowu, E. B. (1973, reprinted 1991) *African Traditional Religion A Definition.* Uganda: Fountain Publications

Klein, M. (1946) Notes on Some Schizoid Mechanisms. *International Journal of Psycho-Analysis.* 27: 99–110.

Le Goff, J. (1992 [1985]) *The Medieval Imagination* (Translated by Arthur Goldhammer), Chicago & London: University of Chicago Press.

Meltzer, D. (2019 [1974]). Chapter Eight: The Paranoid-Schizoid and Depressive Positions1. *Adolescence: Talks and Papers* by Donald Meltzer and Martha Harris, 103–116. *Classic Books.* Psychoanalytic Electronic Publishing, ISSN 2472-6982

Miccoli, G. (1990 [1987]) Monks. *The Medieval World.* Ed. Jacques Le Goff, (Tr. Lydia G. Cochrane. London: Collins and Brown Ltd. 37–73.

Ogden, T. H. (2004). The Analytic Third: Implications for Psychoanalytic Theory and Technique. *Psychoanalytic Quarterly*, 73:167–195.

Rey, H. (1994) *Universals of Psychoanalysis in the Treatment of Borderline and Psychotic States: Factors of Space-Time and Language.* London: Free Association Books.

Searles, H. F. (1987 [1960]) *The Nonhuman Environment In Normal Development and in Schizophrenia.* Madison Connecticut: International Universities Press., Inc.

Searles, H. F. (1962) The Differentiation between Concrete and Metaphorical thinking in the Recovering Schizophrenic Patient. *Journal of the American Psychoanalytic Association*, 10:22–49.

Shields, R. (1991) *Places in the Margin: Alternative geographies of modernity.* London: Routledge.

Shreeve, J. (2015) 'Mystery Man'. *National Geographic.* 228. 4:30–57.

Shulman Y. & Saroff A. "Imagination for Two" Child Psychotherapy during Coronavirus Outbreak: Building a Space for Play When Space Collapses, *Journal of Infant, Child, and Adolescent Psychotherapy*, ISSN: (Print) (Online) Journal homepage: https://www.tandfonline.com/loi/hicp2 Routledge

Smart, N. (1971 [1969]) *The Religious Experience of Mankind*, London and Glasgow: Fontana Library.

Stern, D. N. (1985) *The Interpersonal World of the Infant: A View from Psychoanalysis and Developmental Psychology.* New York: Basic Books.

Stringer, C. (25 May 2016) A comment on the 'Early Neanderthal constructions deep in Bruniquel Cave in south western France' [Accessed 25/06/2017] Paper published in Nature. Available on www.nhm.ac.uk

Tally, R. T. (2013) *Spatiality.* Oxford & New York: Routledge.

Winnicott, D W (2002 [1967]) Mirror-role of Mother and Family in Child Development. [First published 1967] *Playing and Reality.* London: Routledge. (1971, reprinted 2002), p. 111–118.

Winship G. and MacDonald S. G. (2018) *The Essentials of Counselling and Psychotherapy in Primary Schools: On Being a Specialist Mental Health Lead In Schools*, London and New York: Routledge.

Wollheim, R. (1969) The Mind and the Mind's Image of Itself. *International Journal of Psycho-Analysis*. 50:209–220.

Wright, D. (2018) Rooms as Replacements for People: The Consulting Room as a Room Object (pp. 251–262). In: *On Replacement – Cultural, Social and Psychological Representations*. Editors: Owen, J. and Segal, N., Palgrave Macmillan

Wright, D., (2019) Spatialisation and the Fomenting of Political Violence (pp. 167–187). In: *Fomenting Political Violence – Fantasy, Language, Media, Action*. Editors: Kruger, S., Figlio, K. and Richards, B., Palgrave Macmillan

Yates, F. (1966, reprinted 2014) *The Art of Memory*. London. Bodley Head.

Chapter 2

Sigmund Freud, Spatialisation, and Rooms

[This chapter contains material from

the book Chapter; Wright, D. (2018) 'Rooms as Replacements for People: The Consulting Room as a Room Object' (pp. 251–262) in 'Psychoanalysis' section of 'On Replacement – Cultural, Social and Psychological Representations', Eds: Jean Owen and Naomi Segal, Switzerland, Palgrave Macmillan. Reproduced with permission of Palgrave Macmillan.]

In Chapter 1, I discuss phenomena that I have observed in the consulting room, not fully explained by current theory, where patients seem to relate to the consulting room at times separately to me in the transference. I discuss examples from historical, anthropological, and previous clinical experience, that I utilise to formulate my hypothetical alternative theory to explain this phenomenon better. In this chapter, I consider Sigmund Freud's writings, showing his relationship with spaces and spatiality. Freud showed intense and repeated use of spatial imagery and he made meanings for specific spatial locations and their relationship to each such as, The Acropolis, Athens, Pompeii, Rome, Notre Dame, Paris, Charing Cross, and Loch Ness. He also made meaning of buildings and objects in those locations, as well as rooms and their contents, including projecting maternal and paternal figures into the spaces of rooms. None of this was theorised. I argue that although Freud's interest in rooms informed his creation of the consulting room as part of the development of psychoanalysis, it seems that something of his interest has been lost, but perhaps still exists without any formal theorizing. There is, for example, an implicit spatial concern in contemporary psychoanalysis, which is also a root idea for various areas of Psychoanalytic thinking. This considers spatiality in dreams, obsessionality, and hysteria, as well as spatialisation in Freud's conceptualisation of projection as an unformed internal pressure of instinct put into external form, which is necessarily spatial. Formulations of Psychoanalysis have retained spatialising as an unconscious element, and

DOI: 10.4324/9781003188117-2

I wish to bring it to the fore in this study regarding the physical space of the consulting room and its role in the therapeutic process.

The question of why spatialising has been little theorised, including by Freud, is both a 'background' question to this study and also intrinsic to the need for doing the study and the position it takes up in the literature. Why would Freud, who showed such great spatial concerns throughout his life and work, including in his approach to the filling up and usage of his own consulting room, not theorise about that? The answer to that, which I will address in this chapter, is surely an underpinning factor to the relatively unconscious position that the consulting room has continued to take up in its role in the therapeutic process.

Freud's Theory of Instincts – Utilised to Build my Conceptualisation of the Term 'Spatialisation'

Freud suggests in his cultural theories in *Totem and Taboo*: 'It is not to be supposed that men were inspired to create their first system of the universe by pure speculative curiosity. The practical need for controlling the world around them must have played its part.' (Freud, 1955[1913], p. 78). Freud (1957[1915]) also observes that thoughts and feelings that cannot be contained or controlled within the self, need to be projected outside it, where they might be controlled through physical manipulation. In this context, two aspects become particularly relevant. First, there is the projective creation of space which either represents instincts, as I will show in Freud's model, or represents objects, in Object-relations theory, as I show in Chapter 3. Second, there is the manipulation and control of the space with its objects, giving this representation meaning. Freud wrote that internal instinctual stimuli make 'demands on the nervous system and cause it to undertake involved and interconnected activities by which the external world is so changed as to afford satisfaction to the internal source of stimulation' (Freud, 1957[1915], p. 120). These 'interconnected activities' thus combine to form the mechanism of 'spatialisation' – activities in the external world that bring about change externally, so as to 'afford satisfaction' to the instincts internally, while simultaneously providing a representation of the internal world in the material one. I am using Freud's concept of the mechanism and function of projection as a model for the re-presentation of internal need and demand in an external form, where it can be managed and brought into line with satisfactions through the external world. This spatialising is 'the manner in which the process of mastering stimuli takes place' (Freud, 1957[1915], p. 120). Freud writes that '[t]he object of an instinct is the thing in regard to which or through which the instinct is able to achieve its aim' and that this object 'becomes assigned to it only in consequence of being peculiarly fitted to make satisfaction possible' (Freud, 1957[1915], p. 122). Thus, spatialisation is a mechanism that simultaneously involves a psychological projection of meaning and physically acting upon the environment, utilised to master the undifferentiated, relentless, internal pressure of instinct. To spatialise means to manipulate things in the physical world, so as to make an initial projection come true and flesh out a psychologically required meaning.

Additionally, Freud wrote about space being fashioned by projection, after observing that some of his patients manifested their unconscious feelings spatially. He called these manifestations 'mnemic symbols':

> Their symptoms are residues and mnemic symbols of particular (traumatic) experiences. We may perhaps obtain a deeper understanding of this kind of symbolism if we compare them with other mnemic symbols in other fields. The monuments and memorials with which large cities are adorned are also mnemic symbols. [...] [W]hat should we think of a Londoner who paused to-day in deep melancholy before the memorial of Queen Eleanor's funeral [...] or [...] a Londoner who shed tears before the Monument that commemorates the reduction of his beloved metropolis to ashes [...]? Yet every single hysteric and neurotic behaves like these two unpractical Londoners. Not only do they remember painful experiences of the remote past, but they still cling to them emotionally.
>
> (Freud, 1957[1910], pp. 16–17)

Freud also writes of the placing of several of these memorials on a kind of mourning path. Memorials are structures in places and internally structured. What Freud finds, is the monuments are the products of a marking out of space – the creation of a physical representation of an emotional state (which I discuss further in Chapter 8). He utilises these creations as exemplifications of mnemic symbols. These symbols are objects in space, into which feelings are not only projected but which are, in turn, constitutive of these feelings in the first place. Freud describes these mnemic symbols with diagrams (see Fig. 2.1): 'there lies a second system which transforms the momentary excitations of the first system into permanent traces. The schematic picture of our psychical apparatus would then be as follows' (Freud, 1953[1900], p. 538).

The greater our need for containment that cannot be met by our significant others, the higher a perceived threat and the greater the pressure of internal instincts, the less we will be able to think and the more this primitive form of functioning, which I am calling spatialisation, will become utilised. Projection recasts and develops the internal world into the dimensional form of the external world, and in doing so it also creates the objects the ego finds, into which internal unease can be projected.

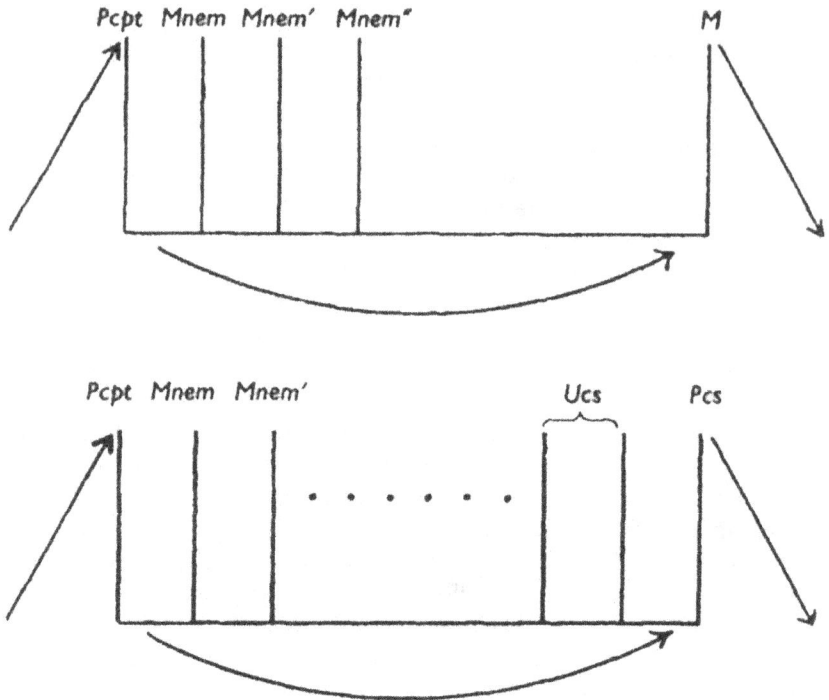

Figure 2.1 Sigmund Freud's diagrams of Mnemic symbols.

Freud and Primary Spatialised Room Transference, Introjected and Re-projected, Re-spatialised (Untheorized): Freud's Rooms

In this section, I suggest that Freud's fascination with the control, ordering, denoting meaning to, writing about, and making diagrams of the interiors of the rooms he inhabited (which I give examples of), is not only a spatialising activity but that it also relates to my Room-object Spatial Matrix (which I will discuss the formulation of next in Chapter 3), *Stage 2 – Room-object*, as he transferred maternal and paternal figures into room spaces. In addition, the *Stage 2 – Room-object* can be re-spatialised into other room spaces, including the consulting room (stages 3 and 4 of the Room-object Spatial Matrix). I show that Freud does this, and I discuss why this was not theorised about in Freud's invention of the consulting room or in his concept of transference.

My first example of a diagram of Freud's, of a room in which he lived or worked, is in Freud's letter of April 5th 1876, to Eduard Silberstein. Freud wrote about the Zoologische Station in Trieste with a map (see Fig. 2.2) and

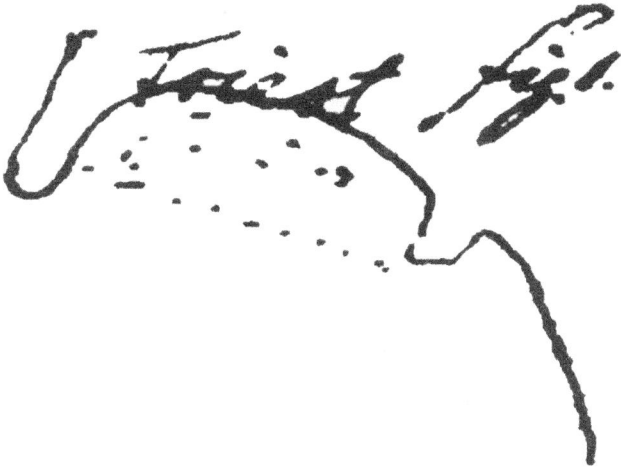

Figure 2.2 Map of Trieste, where Sigmund Freud's room in "Zoologische Station" was located, 1876. Drawing by S. Freud.

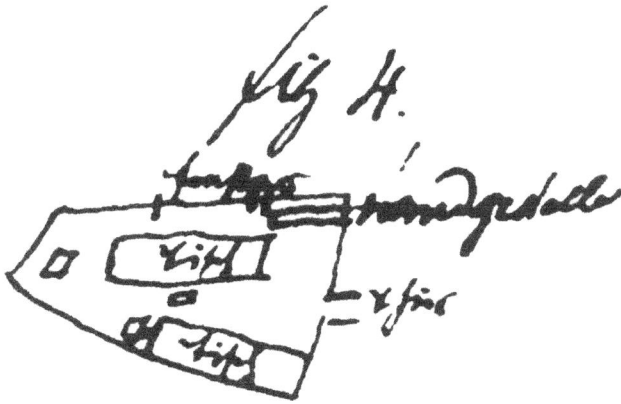

Figure 2.3 Drawing of Sigmund Freud's room in "Zoologische Station" in Trieste, 1876. Drawing by S. Freud.

description of the location of his room where 'the Adriatic is beautiful indeed. Trieste, as you know, lies within a small bay [Fig. 1] [here Fig. 2.2], [...] 'the sea, which may be seen at all times from my window, is usually as smooth as glass.' (Freud, 1990[1876], p. 142). He then gave a detailed account of the interior and spatial array of objects in it (see Fig. 2.3), as well as his desk (see Figs. 2.4 and 2.5), and the objects on it as well as his chair (see Figs 2.4 and 2.6):

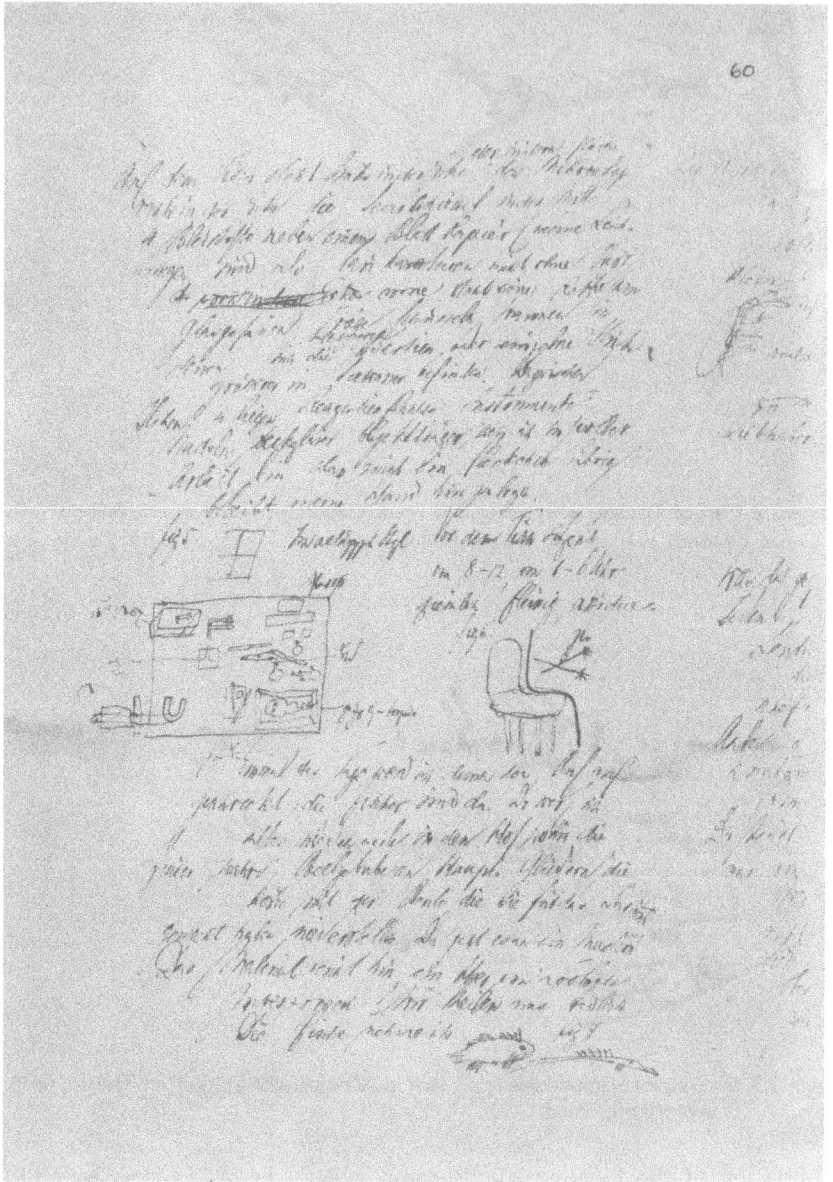

Figure 2.4 Page of Letter from Sigmund Freud to Eduard Silberstein April 5th 1876, showing Freud's drawings of his desk and chair.

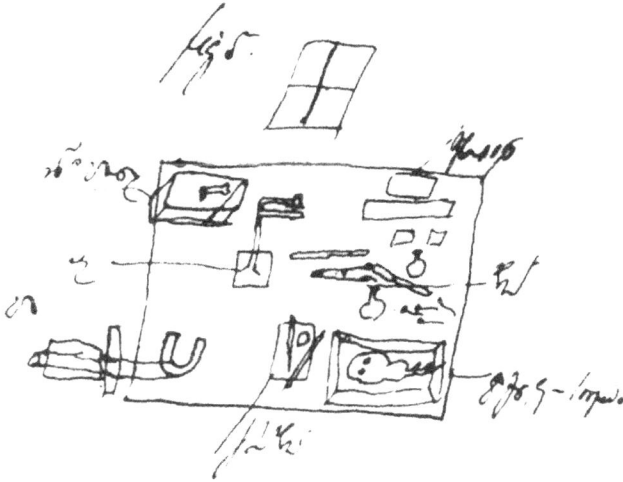

Figure 2.5 Drawing of Sigmund Freud's table in his room in "Zoologische Station" in Trieste, 1876. Drawing by S. Freud.

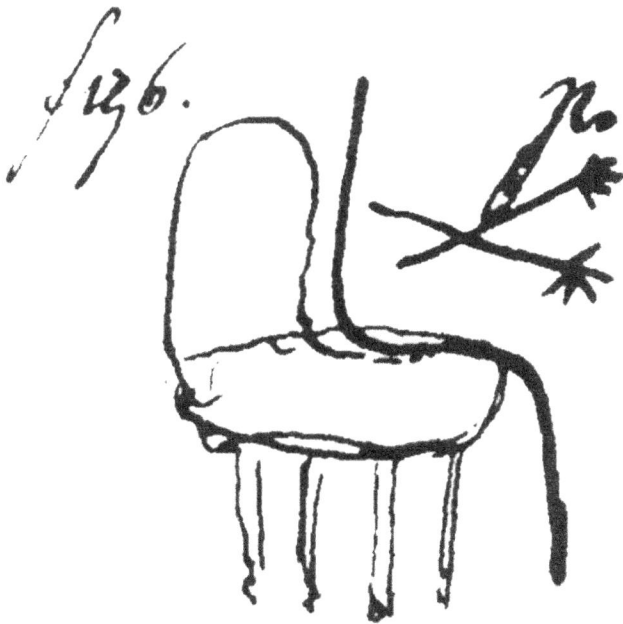

Figure 2.6 Drawing of Sigmund Freud's chair in his room in "Zoologische Station" in Trieste, 1876. Drawing by S. Freud.

My little room has an odd floor plan, one window, in front of which is my work table, with a great number of drawers and a large top, a second table for books and ancillary implements, three chairs, and several shelves holding some twenty test tubes. Last but not least, there is also a sizeable door, which, if you follow its lead, takes you outside [Fig. 4]. [here Fig. 15]. On the left side of the table, in the corner, stands the microscope, in the right corner the dissection dish, in the centre four pencils next to a sheet of paper (my drawings are therefore cartoons, and not without value), in front stands a series of glass vessels, pans, bowls [...] so that when I am busy working there is not a spot left on which I can rest my hand [Fig. 5] [here Fig. 2.5]. I sit at this table from eight to twelve and from one to six, working quite diligently [Fig. 6]. [here Fig. 2.6]

(Freud, 1990[1876], p. 146)

The next example is from Freud's letter to Martha Bernays (October 5th 1883) from the Dermatological Department of the General Hospital, 'he described and sketched his new room and his furniture' (Freud, Freud & Grubrich-Simitis, 1998[1978], p. 104) (see Fig. 2.7).

Ernest Jones wrote a translation:

The 'animal' part of this cavern which fits me as well as a snail-shell fits the snail, is fairly successful, the 'vegetative' part (i.e., the one intended for the ordinary functions of life in opposition to the higher 'animal' functions like writing, reading or thinking) rather less so. [...] Space is in the smallest hut for the lonely longing one.

(Freud, Freud & Grubrich-Simitis, 1998[1978], p. 327)

So here it can be seen that Freud was dividing the room into parts related to physical and psychological functions, as well as evaluating the size of the space depending on the emotional state of the person within it. It might be considered that the dividing of physical and psychological happened in the creation of the consulting room and that the psychological aspects of psychoanalytic technique were theorised (and 'successful') whereas the physical aspects of the room were not theorised about and therefore we could say did not appear 'successful'.

In the next example, shown in a letter of 1882 to his fiancée, Martha Bernays, Freud significantly shows projections of male and female figures into and onto the walls of his room and the spatial array of objects within it (see my Fig. 2.8):

My precious, most beloved girl I knew it was only after you had gone that I would realize the full extent of my happiness and, alas! the degree of my loss as well. I still cannot grasp it, and if that elegant little box and that sweet picture were not lying in front of me, I would think it was all

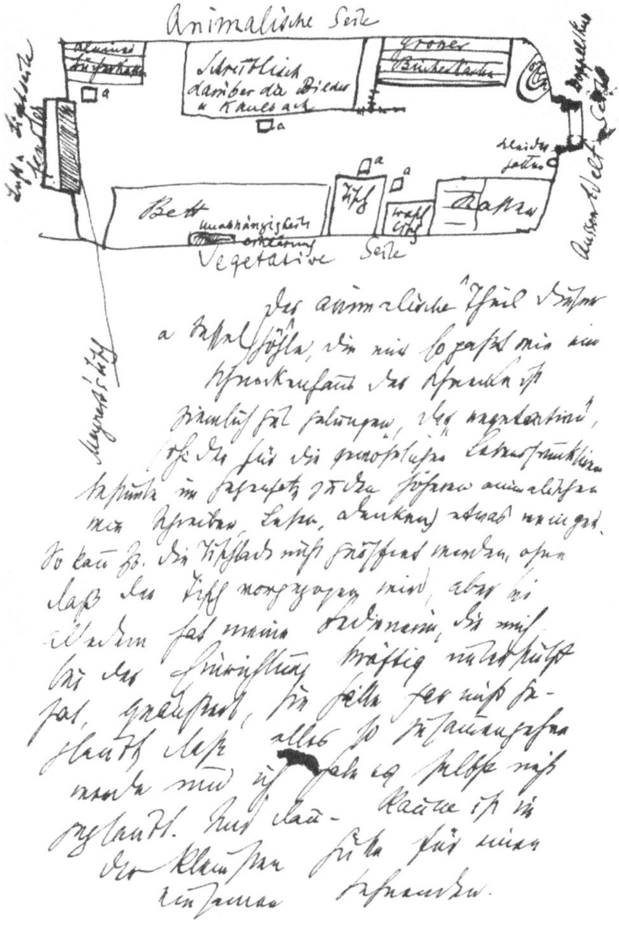

Figure 2.7 Drawing of Sigmund Freud's room in The General Hospital in Vienna, October, 1883. Drawing by S. Freud.

a beguiling dream and be afraid to wake up […] I would so much like to give the picture a place among my household gods that hang above my desk, but while I can display the severe faces of the men I revere, the delicate face of the girl I have to hide and lock away. It lies in your little box and I hardly dare confess how often during the past twenty-four hours I have locked my door and taken it out to refresh my memory.

(Freud, 1961[1882], p. 8)

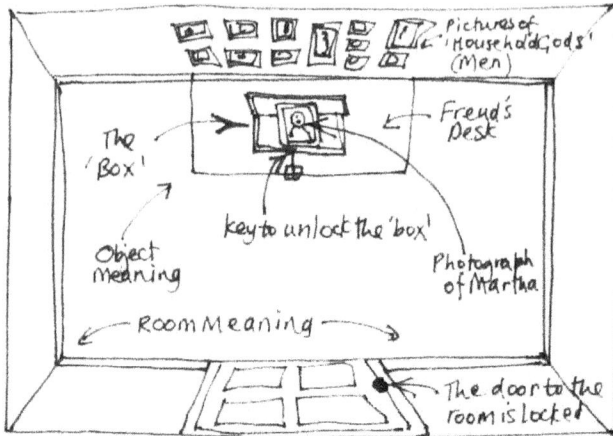

Figure 2.8 An aerial view of Freud's room, 1882. Drawing by D. Wright.

I am suggesting this relates to my hypothetical Room-object Spatial Matrix, *Stage 2 – Primary Spatialised Room Transference*, as he transferred maternal and paternal figures into room spaces, projected onto the walls and objects of the room. Within the scenario in the letter, we can see a possible projection of the father in the pictures of 'household gods' (men) and the 'box' and 'lock' represents the mother, women, and/or Martha relating to the space of the mother's body.

Mother and Women Spatialised Into Rooms, Introjected and Re-projected

I am suggesting that the box and lock metaphors relate to mother and female projection onto the space and objects of that room. The lock metaphor is mentioned again in a letter to Martha on August 18th 1882. In Freud's description of his fantasy of an ideal home that they could have, and the meaning of the furniture, and objects in it. Again, here we have meaning attributed to the spatial array (phantasy) of the home space and control and meaning attributed to the space:

> it occurs to me that we would need two or three little rooms to live and eat in and to receive a guest, and a stove in which the fire for our meals never goes out. And just think of all the things that have got to go into the rooms! Tables and chairs, beds, mirrors, […] pictures on the wall, glasses […], and an enormous bunch of keys – which must make a rattling noise. And there will be so much to enjoy, the books and the sewing table and the cosy lamp, and everything must be kept in good

order or else the housewife, who has divided her heart into little bits, one for each piece of furniture, will begin to fret. [...] And of course we will have to go on telling each other every day that we still love each other. There is something terrible about two human beings who love each other and can find neither the means nor the time to let the other know [...]. If they are left untouched for too long, they diminish imperceptibly or the lock gets rusty; they are there all right but one cannot make use of them.

(Freud, 1961[1882], pp. 27, 28)

Here, Martha is to divide up her heart to attach it to each part of the spatial array of the room and its furniture and objects. This is not dissimilar to the way in which Freud was treating the rooms he lived and worked in, in previous letters, with the furniture and objects labelled (see Figs. 15, 16, and 17). However, in this example with Martha, as with the previous example (Fig. 18) there is a female projection, but because of the introjection and re-spatialisation, in the Room-object Spatial stages to which I refer, the body is also constructed from the phantasy relating to the various objects in rooms, here onto the furniture, and there is also the box and lock metaphor. Freud refers to their relationship as a 'lock', this seems to be a sexual reference, and it is also an echo of the locked 'box' and the locked door, in order to look in the 'box', in his letter to her of two months earlier (Fig. 18). Boxes are a common metaphor for Freud, 'the English 'box' was related to the German 'Büchse' ['receptacle'], [...] 'Bückse' is used as a vulgar term for the female genitals' (Freud, 1953[1900], p. 154). Freud wrote about the possible meaning of a box within the analytic work in the case of Dora where she;

brought out a small ivory box, ostensibly in order to refresh herself with a sweet. She made some efforts to open it, and then handed it to me so I might convince myself how hard it was to open. I expressed my suspicion that the box must mean something special [...]. The box – [in German] [...] was once again only a substitute [...] for the female genitals. There is a great deal of symbolism of this kind in life, but as a rule we pass it by without heeding it.

(Freud, 1953[1905(1901)], p. 77)

Freud also uses the metaphor of a house: 'the dwelling-house was a substitute for the mother's womb, the first lodging, for which in all likelihood man still longs, and in which he was safe and felt at ease' (Freud, 1961[1930], p. 91) and of a room, '[i]t seems to me more likely that a room became the symbol of a woman as being the space which encloses human beings' (Freud, 1963[1916], p. 163). Freud also reported a dream of his mother, involving wardrobes and cupboards:

I saw myself standing in front of a cupboard ['Kasten'] demanding
something and screaming [...]. Then suddenly my mother, looking
beautiful and slim, walked into the room [...]. I had missed my mother,
and had come to suspect that she was shut up in this wardrobe or cupboard
[...]. The wardrobe or cupboard was a symbol [...] of [...] mother's inside.

(Freud, 1960[1901], pp. 49–51)

Freud's mother had just given birth to his sister. This dream resonates with
his case study of 'Little Hans', where Hans describes the spatial manifestation of his unprocessed feelings about the birth of his sister, according
to Freud, when Hans refers to boxes transported on carts (see Fig. 2.9).

The boxes represent his mother's womb with the baby sister. 'We can now
recognize that all furniture-vans and drays and buses were only stork-box
carts, and were only of interest to Hans as being symbolic representations of
pregnancy; and that when a heavy or heavily loaded horse fell down he can
have seen in it only one thing – a childbirth, a delivery' (Freud, 1955[1909],
p. 128). In the same way, Freud's mother emerges 'beautiful and slim' from
the cupboard. A greater insight into Freud's dream about his mother can
perhaps be gained from Joseph Berke's observation that Freud experienced
his mother as 'emotionally unavailable' and, we might think, possibly
physically less available. He writes:

Amalie became pregnant again with her second son, Julius. This baby
also carried the same name as Amalie's brother and beloved companion.
Baby Julius died when Sigmund was two years old from an infection
and Amalie's brother passed on at around the same time from
tuberculosis. Both losses left his mother heartbroken and emotionally
unavailable to Sigmund.

(Berke, 2015, p. xiii)

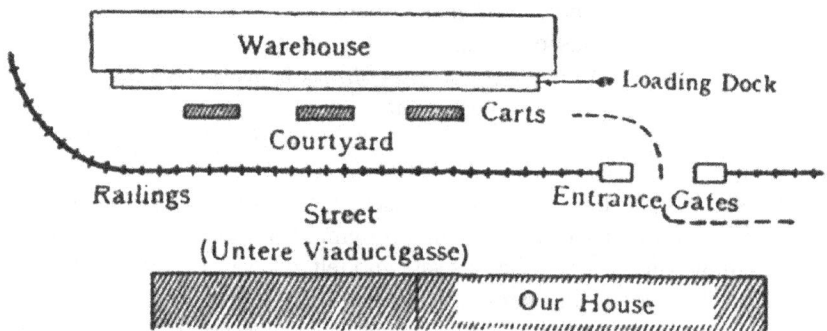

Figure 2.9 'Little Hans is specially frightened when carts drive into or out of the yard'
(Freud 1955[1909]).

This may give us an insight into Freud's fascination with rooms. Rooms may represent the mother or a replacement of her care when she is absent emotionally and/or physically. Another room of significance for Freud was the 'cabinet' he was given when his family moved to a larger flat in 1875, when he was 19:

> The 'cabinet', a long and narrow room separated from the rest of the flat, with a window looking onto the street, was allotted to Sigmund; it contained a bed, chairs, shelf, and writing-desk. There he lived and worked until he became an *interne* at the hospital; all through the years of his school and university life the only thing that changed in it was an increasing number of crowded book-cases. In his teens he would even eat his evening meal there so as to lose no time from his studies. He had an oil lamp to himself, while the other bedrooms had only candles.
>
> (Jones, 1967[1953], pp. 45–46)

Here Freud was given a special room, unlike his siblings, who had to share rooms, and it also featured special objects. Perhaps the room represented a special time of just him and mother – it was a room for just him. I suggest that this may be the original site of spatialisation (Room-spatialisation) which was introjected and re-projected into the rooms we have looked at, such as the General Hospital (see Fig. 2.7), and the Zoologische Station in Trieste (Fig. 2.3). These are the first rooms he lived in after leaving home, where he may have re-projected his projection into the 'cabinet', which he may have substituted for the role of mother. Before Freud invented the concepts of transference or the consulting room, he transferred the meaning of people onto the space of a room and the objects within it. Freud wrote of a dream relating to the stairway leading to his consulting room: 'That night I had the following dream: I was very incompletely dressed and was going upstairs from a flat on the ground floor to a higher storey [...] [m]y consulting-room and study are on the upper ground floor (Freud, 1900, p. 238). Later Freud goes into more detail about architectural metaphor in 'The Genitals Represented by Buildings, Stairs and Shafts', where he writes that in relation to stairs 'from my own knowledge derived elsewhere that climbing down, like climbing up in other cases, described sexual intercourse in the vagina'. (Freud, 1900, p. 365) So, there is a female reference of going up into his consulting room, perhaps like his reference to the womb (see p. 39). In this section, we looked at Freud's projection of maternal and female figures (or mother function) and we now go on to look at Freud's projection of paternal/masculine figures, as well as, again, into his consulting room.

Father and 'Gods' Spatialised Into Rooms and Locations

Returning to Freud's letter to Martha of 1882 (Fig. 2.8), in which we have looked at his female projections, I will now look at male aspects. Freud writes of 'my household gods that hang above my desk [...] display the severe faces of the men I revere' (Freud, 1961[1882], p. 8).

These are perhaps male family members as well as other men that he reveres on the walls of the room. I suggest that the significance of Charcot, who may have fulfilled a father-like role for Freud, or even an idealised father, was incorporated into Freud's consulting room. Freud hung a picture of Charcot in his Consulting room, which is a black and white print (see Fig. 2.10) of an engraving by Eugene Pirodon after the oil painting by Pierre Aristide André Brouillet entitled 'A Clinical Lesson at the Salpêtrière' (1887) which shows Charcot demonstrating hypnosis on the Salpêtrière patient, Marie "Blanche" Wittmann.

Freud hung the print in his consulting room in Berggasse 19, left of the door, above the shelves, as can be seem in this photograph by Edmund Engelman (Fig. 2.11). Freud later, on moving to his room in Maresfield

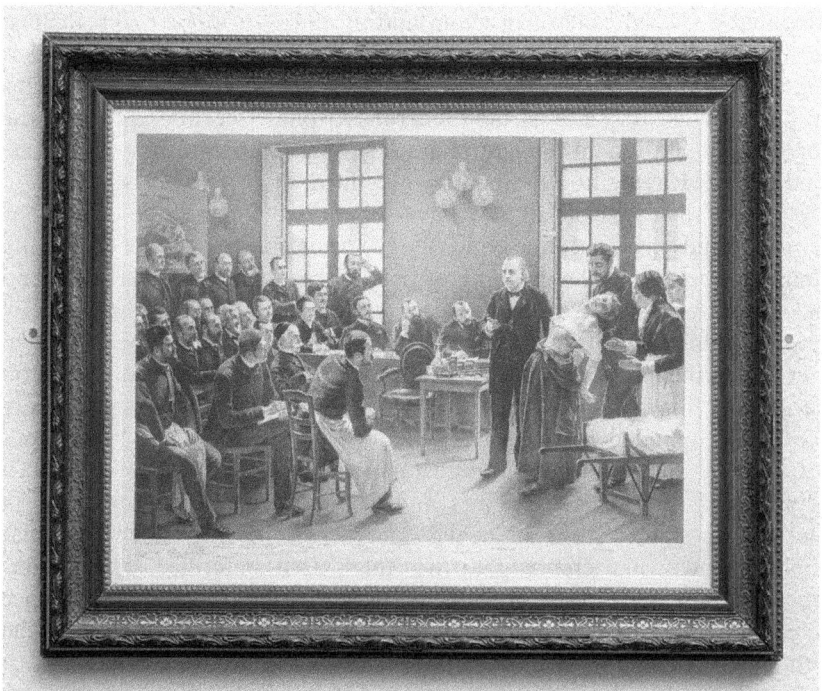

Figure 2.10 Engraving by Eugene Pirodon, of the oil painting by Pierre Aristide André Brouillet, entitled 'A Clinical Lesson at the Salpêtrière' (1887) which hung in Sigmund Freud's consulting rooms in Berggasse 19 and Maresfield Gardens.

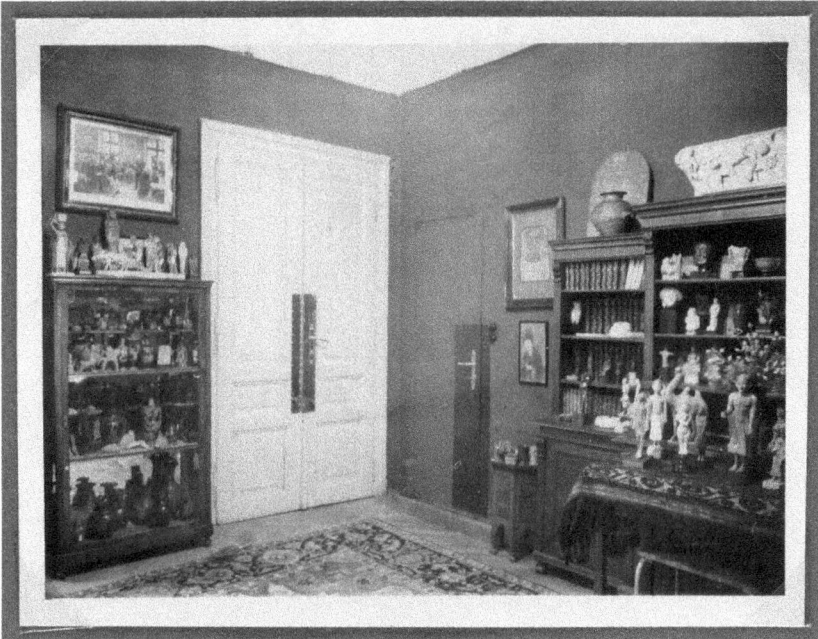

Figure 2.11 Photograph by Edmund Engleman, 1938, showing engraving by Eugene Pirodon of the oil painting by Pierre Aristide André Brouillet entitled 'A Clinical Lesson at the Salpêtrière' (1887), hanging in Sigmund Freud's consulting rooms in Berggasse 19, on the top left side of the photograph.

Gardens, placed it in the central and important position in the consulting room, above the couch (see Fig. 2.12, top right corner).

In a letter to Martha on November 24th 1885 Freud wrote about being a student of Charcot:

> I am really very comfortably installed now and I think I am changing a great deal. I will tell you in detail what is affecting me. Charcot, who is one of the greatest of physicians and a man whose common sense borders on genius, is simply wrecking all my aims and opinions. I sometimes come out of his lectures as from out of Nôtre Dame, with an entirely new idea about perfection.
>
> (Freud, 1961[1885], pp. 184–185)

Here he uses his meaning of the building (Notre Dame) to represent something of his feelings about Charcot which for him, represent 'as an entirely new ideas about perfection'. This is a complex set of symbols layered up. Ernest Jones writes of Freud's relationship to Paris and Notre Dame;

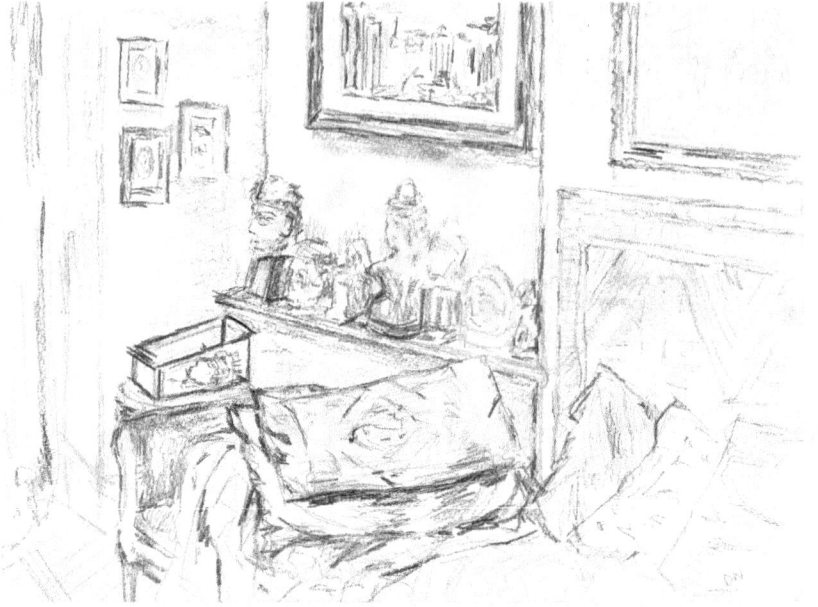

Figure 2.12 Drawing of Maresfield Gardens showing the engraving of the Charcot painting above the couch (top right). Drawing by D. Wright.

Of his life in Paris as a student of Charcot's in the winter of 1885–6, Freud had so much to say […]. The very name of the city had a magic. […] Freud wrote: 'Paris had been for many years the goal of my longings, and the bliss with which I first set foot on its pavements I took as a guarantee that I should attain the fulfilment of other wishes also.' […] [U]ndoubtedly the building that most impressed him in Paris was Notre-Dame. It was the first time in his life that he had the feeling of being inside a church. He mentioned climbing the tower on two occasions […]. He entered into the spirit of Victor Hugo's *Notre-Dame* […] and even said he preferred it to neuropathology. His choice of souvenir of Paris was a photograph of Notre-Dame.

(Jones, 1967[1953], pp. 171–172)

Notre-Dame as a space became important in itself for Freud, within the spatial array of Paris that has a 'magic' spatial manifestation of the idea that he will fulfil his wishes there, which he also related to Charcot, representing his interactions with Charcot and the feelings of 'perfection'. He shows his feelings for a person (Charcot) equated with his feelings for a space (Notre Dame) which is then re-projected on to the wall of the consulting room. This relates to what I am calling Room-spatialisation. In hanging Charcot on his consulting room wall, Freud was bringing something of his feeling about Charcot and his feeling of Notre Dame 'an entirely new idea about perfection', (Freud, 1961[1885], p. 185) into the room. This related to Charcot's 'genius' and him being an idealised paternal figure, spatialised onto (and placed on in the form of the lithograph) the walls off the consulting room, perhaps to imbue the consulting room with these qualities, like the 'household gods' he 'revered' in Fig. 18, perhaps affording protection, assistance or 'perfection'. I now look further at representations relating to paternal projections (relating to his father) spatialised in the consulting room.

Freud's Consulting Room, Transference, and Spatialisation

Freud had many objects in the consulting room associated with classical Rome and Greece which I suggest incorporate meanings projected relating to Freud's Father. Freud describes the meaning and act of sitting on the Acropolis and how it relates to his feelings about his Father: 'The very theme of Athens and the Acropolis in itself contained evidence of the son's superiority. Our father had been in business, he had had no secondary education, and Athens could not have meant much to him' (Freud, 1964[1936], p. 247) and that '[I]t must be that a sense of guilt was attached to the satisfaction in having gone such a long way' (Freud, 1964[1936], p. 247). This contrasts with his description of Charcot and his 'genius'. Freud wrote that Rome represented 'unattainable aims' (Freud, 1953[1900], p. 195), unlike Paris, that promised to fulfil wishes, Freud recounted an experience when his Father told him:

> A Christian came up to me and with a single blow knocked off my cap into the mud and shouted: "Jew! get off the pavement!"' 'And what did you do?' I asked. 'I went into the roadway and picked up my cap,' was his quiet reply. This struck me as unheroic conduct on the part of the big, strong man who was holding the little boy by the hand. I contrasted this situation with another which fitted my feelings better: the scene in which Hannibal's father, Hamilcar Barca, made his boy swear before the household altar to take vengeance on the Romans. Ever since that time Hannibal had had a place in my phantasies.
>
> (Freud, 1953[1900], p. 197)

Here there is something else paternal represented, something flawed, imperfect, unheroic, different from Hannibal, as a boy, at the 'household altar' and contrasting with his own 'household gods' which alongside the Charcot's image on the wall looking down as the men he 'reveres'. He had many objects from classical Rome and Greece which may contain some of that meaning for him (see Figs. 2.11 to 2.16). Eugene Victor Walter wrote that 'Edmund Engleman, who photographed Freud's household [...] reports

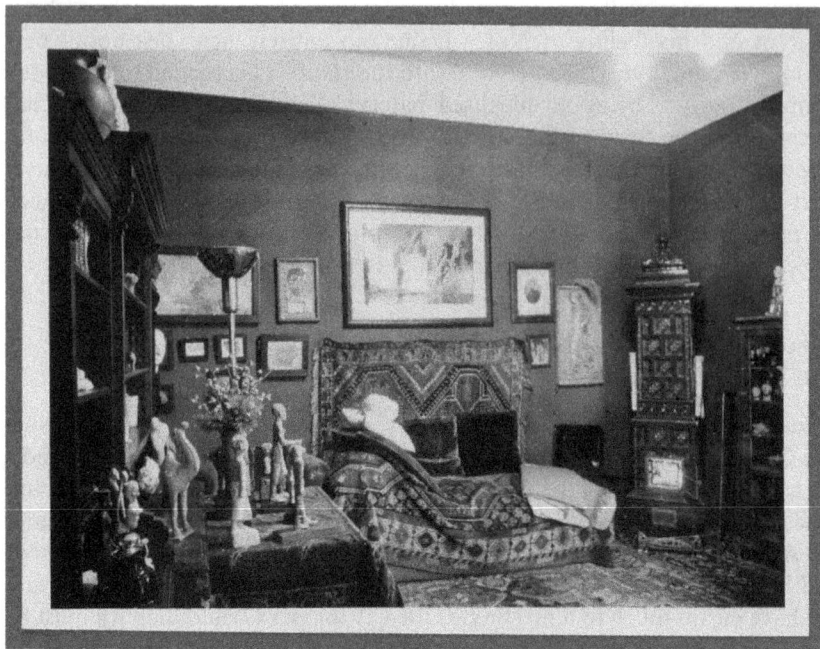

Figure 2.13 Photograph of Sigmund Freud's consulting room in Vienna, May 1938. Photograph by E. Engleman.

his impressions: "Antiquities filled every available spot in the (consulting) room. I was overwhelmed by the masses of figurines which overflowed every surface".' (Walter, 1988, p. 103). Engleman took the photographs (see Figs. 2.11, 2.13, & 2.14) in 1938, shortly before the Freud moved to London and his rooms were dismantled and packed up to send everything to London. Arnold Werner describes how; 'August Aichorn, an intimate of Freud, knew Engleman as a young, innovative photographer [...]. Aware of Freud's imminent departure from Vienna, Aichorn was concerned that a visual re-cord be established of the setting in which Freud had worked and lived since 1891.' (Werner, 2002, p. 445) and goes on to describe how; 'Most of the photographs in the book are part of an exhibit [...] some of the photographs can be seen at the Freud museums in London [three of which are shown here, Figs 2.11, 2.13, & 2.14 © Freud Museum London] and Vienna [...]. The exhibit photographs are printed from the original negatives and are as large as 24 × 24 inches. At this size, their quality is immediately apparent. One is placed in the midst of Freud's collection of antiquities that covered nearly every surface, and artwork that covered all of the walls.' (Werner, 2002, p. 447). As Engleman puts it 'the masses of figurines which overflowed every surface' (Walter, 1988, p. 103). This is reminiscent of Freud's own

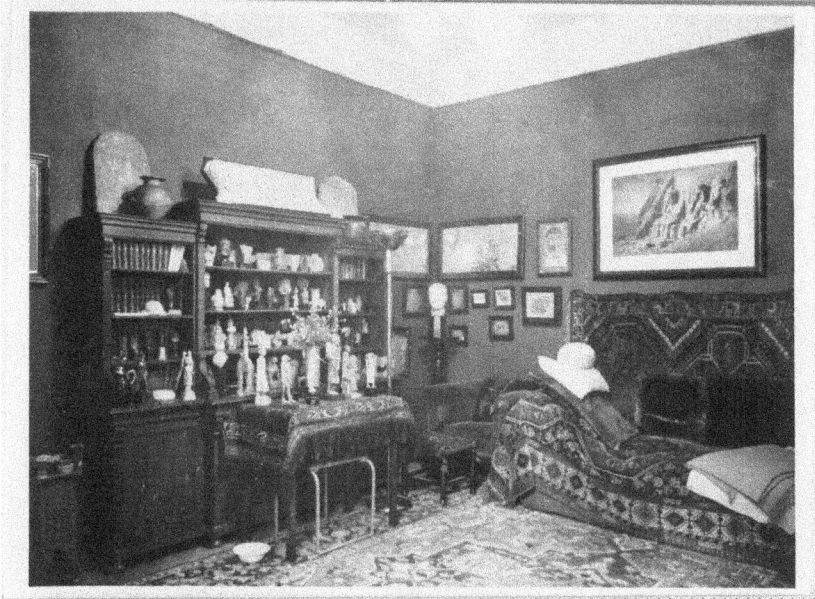

Figure 2.14 Photograph of Sigmund Freud's consulting room in Vienna, May 1938. Photograph by E. Engleman.

description of his desk in his room in Zoologische Station in Trieste, 1876 (see Fig. 2.5) where 'there is not a spot left on which I can rest my hand' (Freud, 1990[1876], p. 146), here however it is not a microscope, dissection dish and glass vessels but some of his 'over 2000 antiquities' that Ro Spankie mentions (Spankie, 2015, Back-cover), which relate to the 'house hold gods' (Freud, 1961[1882], p. 8) that he describes.

Freud also uses Rome as an example of his theory of the mechanisms of memory:

> in mental life nothing which has once been formed can perish [...]. We will choose as an example the history of the Eternal City. Historians tell us that the oldest Rome was the *Roma Quadrata*, a fenced settlement on the Palatine. [...] [W]e will ask ourselves how much a visitor, whom we will suppose to be equipped with the most complete historical and topographical knowledge, may still find left of these early stages in the Rome of to-day.
>
> (Freud, 1961[1930], p. 69)

Freud had a statue of the Gravida, which Freud wrote of as relating to 'burial by repression and excavation by analysis' (Freud, 1959[1907],

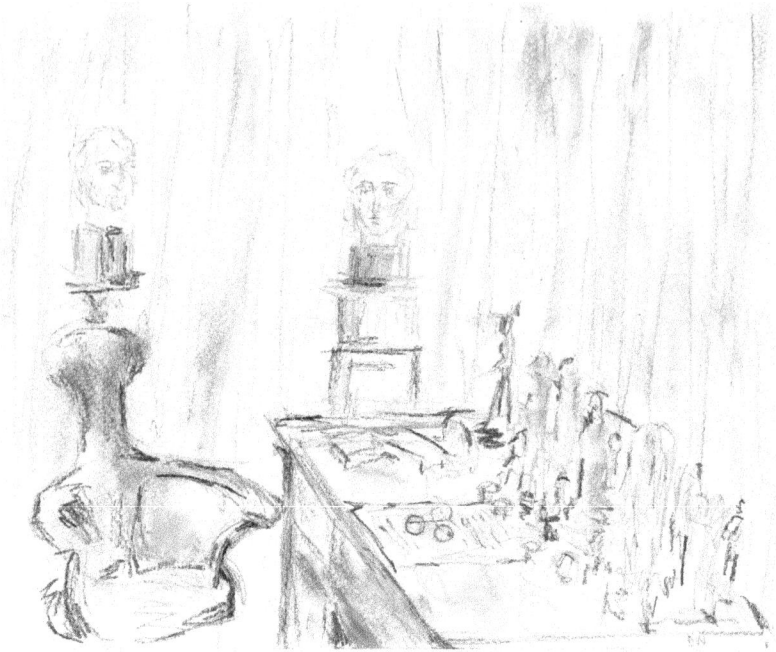

Figure 2.15 Sigmund Freud's room in Maresfield Gardens with his desk, chair, and figures on the desk. Drawing by D. Wright.

pp. 5–18). Freud's patient Pankejeff, 'The Wolfman' wrote; 'Freud himself explained his love for archaeology in that the psychoanalyst, like the archaeologist in his excavations, must uncover layer after layer of the patient's psyche, before coming to the deepest, most valuable treasures.' (Gardiner Ed., 1989[1972], p. 139). So Pankejeff is describing the patient's psyche, much like Freud's description of Rome and memory (1961 [1930]). Freud also had statuettes of Osiris, of which Ro Spankie wrote, 'It has been noted by several commentators that despite having four Osiris figures on his desk, Freud makes no reference to the complex relationship between Osiris and Isis; siblings, lovers and parents, [...] reveals resistances in Freud's self-analysis to traumatic events in his own childhood' (Spankie, 2015, p. 84). There is an idea here that the objects (Osiris) represents something unconscious for Freud, unanalysed and what I would call spatialised. Hilda Doolittle refers to one of the Osiris figures in her account of her analysis with Sigmund Freud: I told him about the little statues or images in the house that Lawrence had first spoken of [...] The Professor [Freud] said, "Come and see if we can find them." We went into

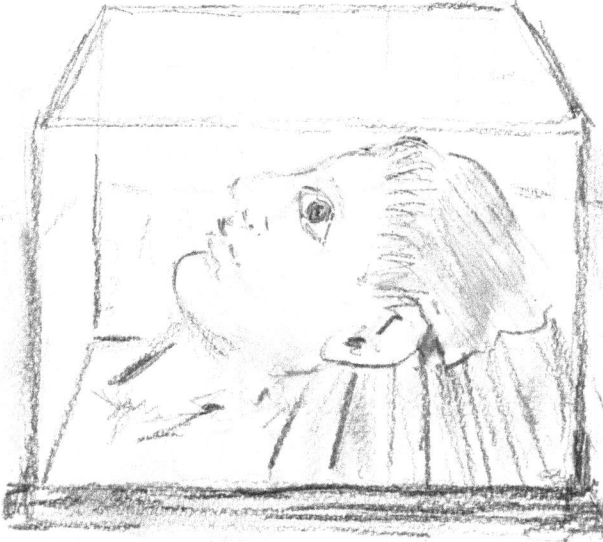

Figure 2.16 Head in glass box in Sigmund Freud's study, Maresfield Gardens. Drawing by D. Wright.

the other room; he brought out various treasures from behind the glass doors. [...] The Professor brought out a wooden Osiris [...]. We went back to the couch.' (Doolittle, 2012 [1956], p. 172). And on another occasion, 'the Professor has gone into the other room to find a new dog to show me. He brings back a broken wooden dog' (Doolittle, 2012[1956], p. 147). Freud was doing something publicly with a patient (Hilda Doolittle), and privately with his feelings about these items and indeed the entire interior of his consulting room. Freud wrote that, 'everything connected with the present situation represents a transference to the doctor.' (Freud, 1955[1913], p. 138). Did he intend for the meaning of his objects to be utilised and connected to him or were the objects, including the entire spatial array of the room and pictures on the walls, also there for his own spatialising usage? Or were they intended for use in the transference for the patient? Could he be missing that the patients may, like him, have their own projections and spatialising relating to his room, in which they also resided, as an experience of their own history of spatialising, separate from him as a transference object? In one of the few texts in which Freud writes about this about this, he writes:

> I am certainly not the first person to have been struck by the resemblance between what are called obsessive actions in sufferers from nervous affections and the observances by means of which believers give expression to their piety. The term 'ceremonial', which has been applied to some of these obsessive actions, is evidence of this [...] they serve important interests of the personality and that they give expression to experiences that are still operative and to thoughts that are cathected with affect. They do this in two ways, either by direct or by symbolic representation; and they are consequently to be interpreted either historically or symbolically [...] The same patient could only sit on one particular chair and could only get up from it with difficulty.
>
> (Freud, 1959 [1907], pp. 117–120)

Here he writes of actions that have an obsessive quality, their purpose (I call spatialising), and of a patient who spatialises about their chair. I am suggesting that this is primitive and pre-transferential. Freud writes on transference that 'the patient sees in his analyst the return – the reincarnation – of some important figure out of his childhood or past, and consequently transfers onto him feelings and reactions which undoubtedly applied to this model. It soon becomes evident that this fact of transference is a factor of undreamt-of importance' (Freud, 1940, p. 52). Freud was doing things within the spatial array of the consulting room with objects, meanings of and arrangements of objects, and what I call spatialising that he at no point theorised about. What was the role that Freud intended his consulting room and its objects to fulfil for his patients in their treatment? Doolittle suggests of Freud's consulting room:

> Inside the Cathedral we find regeneration or reintegration. This room is the Cathedral. [...] The house is home, the house is the Cathedral. He said he wanted me to feel at home here. The house in some indescribable way depends on father – mother. At the point of integration or re-integration, there is no conflict over rival loyalties. The Professor's surroundings and interests seem to derive from my mother rather than from my father, and yet to say the "transference" is to Freud as mother does not altogether satisfy me.
>
> (Doolittle, 2012[1956], p. 146)

So here Doolittle was considering both mother and father in the consulting room which she described as 'cathedral' and 'home'. Doolittle continued with the 'cathedral' metaphor for the consulting room; 'the cathedral of my dream was Sigmund Freud. "No," he said, "not me – but analysis." (Doolittle, 2012[1956], p. 147). Doolittle is writing about transference onto Freud as Father or Mother, but she is also describing a transference onto the consulting room, something like a cathedral, a home. I have been discussing cathedrals and their meanings as a place of common and personal meanings (Westminster Abbey) as well as Freud's association to Notre dame. Similarly, Mahon described the consulting room as the 'house of transference' (Mahon, 2005, p. 29).

I suggest that this model is transferred onto the consulting room which is 'put in the place of' a person or another room. This is like my hypothesised Room-object Spatialisation Matrix -Stage 3- *Secondary Spatialised Room-object in the Consulting Room*. There is a replacement of the person or room with the walls of the consulting room, and that this is also of great 'importance'. I am suggesting that this is part of the role in the consulting room (untheorised about) where the space of the room and its meaning can represent projected feelings about a person to the space of a room and then re-projected into the consulting room, which can be imbued with the original room meaning. Freud did not write a spatial theory for the consulting room- such as Feng Shui (see page 12), that Eastern carpets and pillows, rugs on the walls, objects and so on, as well as the way that they are arrayed, play an active part of the psychic reality for himself and his patients. I suggest that to this day, psychotherapists copy Freud's foreign rug arrangement, either on their walls (behind the couch) or floors as well as couch coverings and cushions. In Mark Gerald's photography project 'In the Shadow of Freud's Couch: Portraits of Psychoanalysts in Their Offices' he wrote 'The Victorian consulting room of Sigmund Freud, with its oriental rug-draped couch, set a mood and technique that governed psychoanalytic life for much of its first century' (Gerald, 2009). In forty-one of Gerald's photographs of psychoanalysts in their consulting room, ten of the photographs of rooms showed eastern rugs. This is a quarter of the rooms. An example of this can be also found in Wayne Myers' case study where he writes that after giving an interpretation to his patient, 'She took one of the Moroccan carpets I have thrown across my couch and wrapped herself in it, as in a swaddling blanket. (Myers, 1994, p. 1167). We identify with Freud and, like him, leave the significance of spatialisation unconscious.

I am suggesting that analysts have copied Freud's original consulting room, as if there were a spatialising system (such as that Feng Shui as discussed on page 12) which Freud created to facilitate efficacious therapeutic work, as if, as Freud wrote:

Miraculous cures properly so-called take place in the case of believers under the influence of adjuncts calculated to intensify religious feelings—that is to say, in places where a miracle-working image is worshipped [...], or where the relics of a saint are preserved as a treasure [...], the reputation of the place and the respect in which it is held act as substitutes for the influence of the group [...]. Where so many powerful forces converge, we need feel no surprise if the goal is sometimes really reached.

(Freud, 1953[1890], pp. 289-290)

Aphasia, the Spatial Layout of the Brain, the Mind, and Rooms

In a letter to Martha of October 9th 1883, Freud wrote:

It seems as though the waves of the great world do not lap against my door; at other times I have to fight against the sensation of being a monk in his cell [...]. Strange creatures are billeted in my brain. Cases, theories, diagnostics, formulas have moved into brain accommodations most of which have been standing empty, the whole of medicine is becoming familiar and fluid to me [...]. When a letter from you arrives the whole dream fades, life enters my cell [...] and gone are the empty theories "according to the present status of science," as they are invariably called. Then the world turns so warm, so gay, so easy to understand. My sweet [...] Oh Marty, it is so much more lovely to be a *human* being than a warehouse for certain monotonous experiences. But one is not allowed to be a human being for an hour unless one has been a machine or a warehouse for eleven hours.

(Freud, 1961[1883], p. 68)

So here in 1883, he is thinking about a cell (small room) which he uses as a metaphor for himself, and the 'accommodation' of the brain, so there is a thinking about where the brain lives, where thinking lives and how Martha (and his connection and feelings towards her) change his 'great emotional and excitable state' when a letter arrives and his thinking. Here we have the beginnings of brain, mind, rooms, and the changing of emotional states.

Freud's diagrams of brain mechanics around this time are reminiscent of his room drawings above, and also to later diagrams of psychological mechanisms all of which have a spatiality of their own. For example, in 'Critical Introduction to Neuropathology' (Freud, 2012[1887] pp. 197–199) he shows the below three diagrams (Figs. 2.17, 2.18, and 2.19). Not only do these seem to relate to the way in which he was treating his rooms, but they also relate to his later diagrams of psychological mechanisms that came after his formulation of psychoanalytic theory.

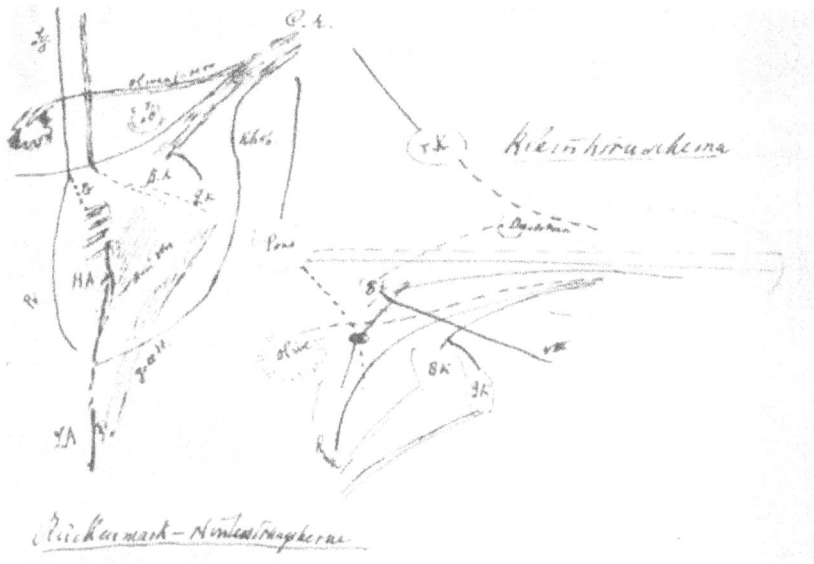

Figure 2.17 Freud's drawing of the brain's workings (originally 'Figure 2. Schema I/a and I/b' p.197). Drawing by S. Freud.

Here are some examples of his diagrams to exemplify psychoanalytic theory below. Note the similarity here of Fig. 2.18 to Fig. 2.20 Freud's 'Schematic Picture of Sexuality' (Freud, 1966[1892], pp. 202–205) as well as 2.3, Freud's room in "Zoologische Station" in Trieste. And likewise, Figs. 2.17 to 2.21. Freud also uses room metaphor in relation to psychoanalytic theory and the brain:

> The crudest idea of these systems is the most convenient for us—a spatial one. Let us therefore compare the system of the unconscious to a large entrance hall, in which the mental impulses jostle one another like separate individuals. Adjoining this entrance hall there is a second, narrower, room—a kind of drawing-room—in which consciousness, too, resides. [...] The impulses in the entrance hall of the unconscious are out of sight of the conscious, which is in the other room; to begin with they must remain unconscious.
>
> (Freud, 1963[1917], p. 295)

In 1923, Freud wrote about the unconscious again, exploring the ego 'spatially', again, with a diagram that looks like one of his room drawings, here representing the workings of the mind:

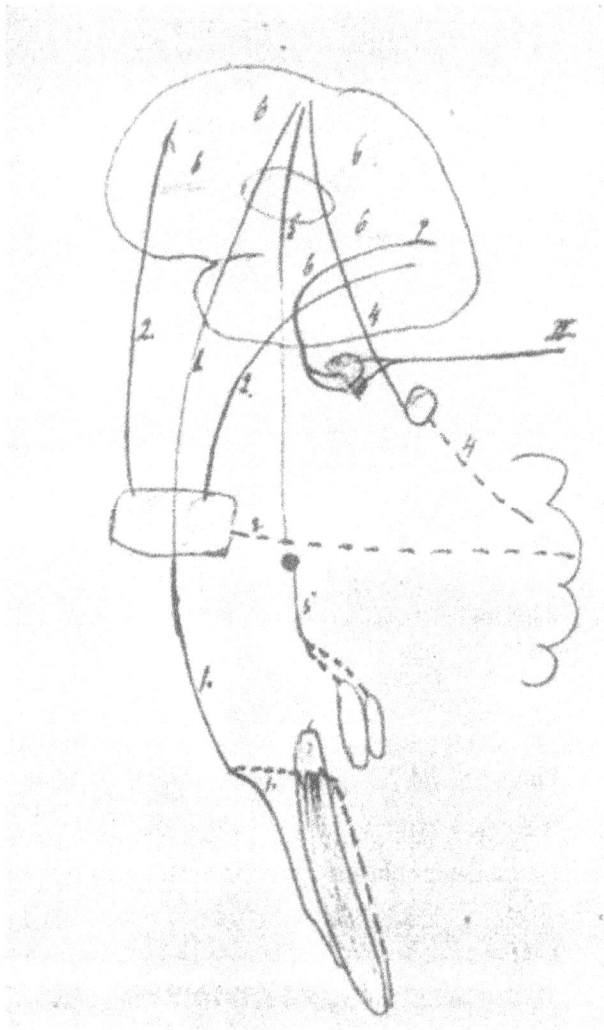

Figure 2.18 Freud's drawing of the brain's workings (originally Figure 3. Schema 2: Tracts of the cerebral grey p.198). Drawing by S. Freud.

We have said that consciousness is the *surface* of the mental apparatus; that is, we have ascribed it as a function to a system which is spatially the first one reached from the external world—and spatially not only in the functional sense but, on this occasion, also in the sense of anatomical dissection [...] The state of things which we have been describing can be represented diagrammatically.

(Freud, 1955[1923], pp. 19–24) [Fig. 2.22]

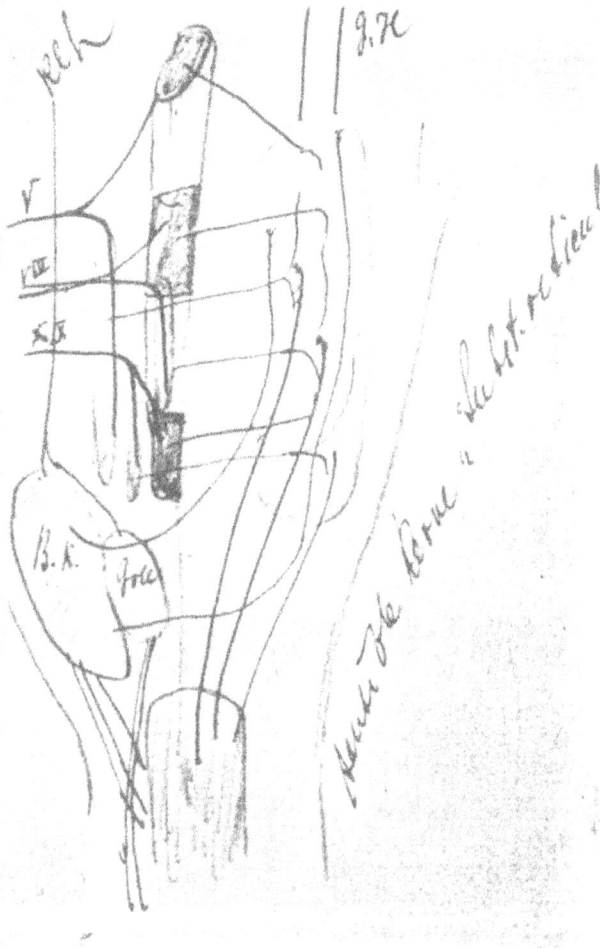

Figure 2.19 Freud's drawing of the brain's workings (originally Figure 4 Schema 3: Sensory nuclei and substantia reticularis p.199). Drawing by S. Freud.

In 'Aphasia, A critical study' Freud wrote that brain – '"localization", i.e., of the restriction of nervous functions to anatomically definable areas, which pervades the whole of recent neuro-pathology' (Freud, 1953 [1891], p. 1), where different functions are located in different parts of the brain, was unfounded. These ideas of brain localization were of great interest generally at the time. This can be seen in the phrenology model (see Fig. 2.23) where the brain is made up of different spaces or spatialized areas.

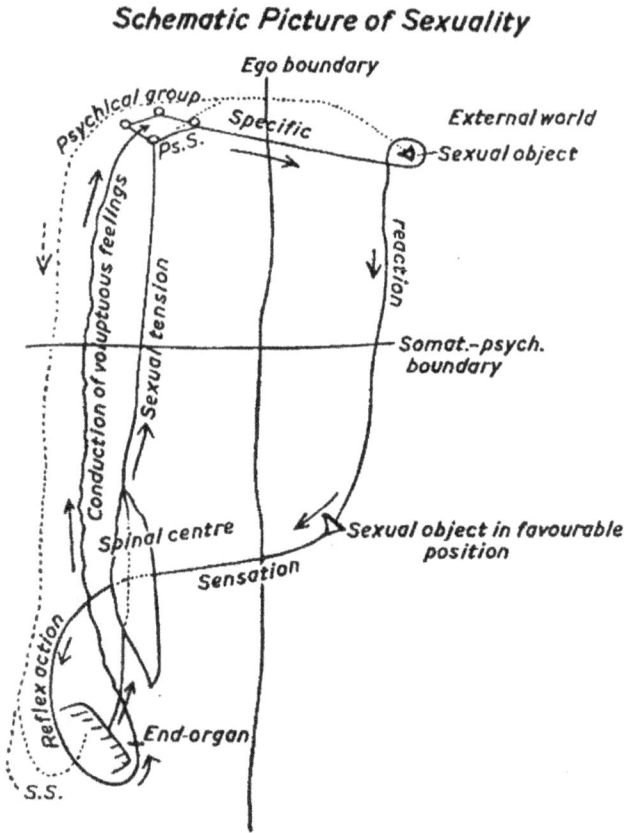

Figure 2.20 Sigmund Freud's Fig 1. 'Schematic Picture of Sexuality'.

Stengel wrote:

Freud's book on aphasia is known to a small circle of experts only. [...] Not only did Freud make valuable contributions to neurology but he laid the foundation of psychoanalysis. It has gradually been recognised in recent years that his anatomical, neurological and psychoanalytical works form a continuum. The book on aphasia demonstrates this clearly. It was the first of the author's studies dealing with mental activities and thus provides a link between the two apparently separate periods in his working life. [...] It appeared when neurologists were intensely preoccupied with the localization of cerebral functions. [...] Freud was the first in the German speaking world to subject the current

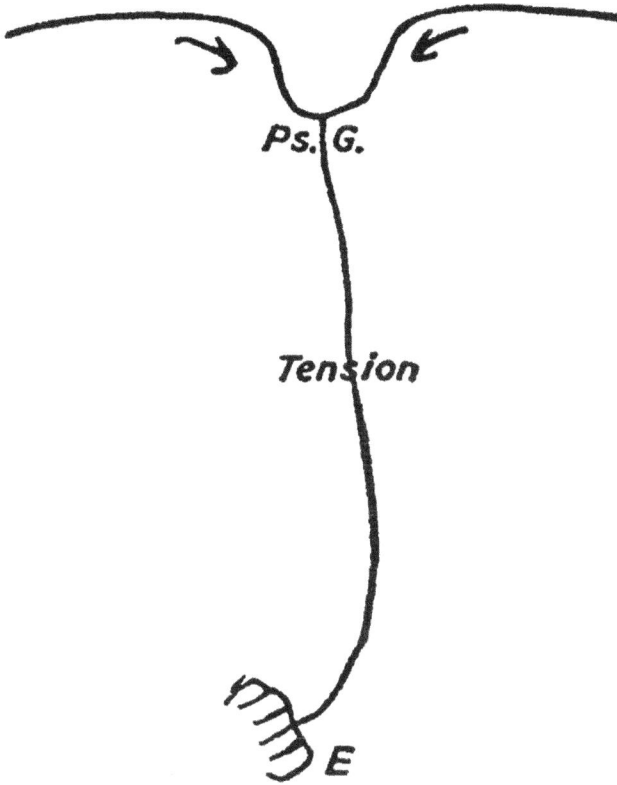

Figure 2.21 Sigmund Freud's Fig 2. 'Schematic Picture of Sexuality'.

theory of localization to a systematic critical analysis. In challenging both a powerful scientific trend and its most influential representatives he showed himself an independent thinker of considerable courage.

(Stengel, in Freud, 1953[1891], pp. ix–x)

Freud's alternative theory to localization was that the brain has an integrating function:

we must not search for the physio-logical substratum of mental activity in this or that part of the brain but we have to regard it as the outcome of processes spread widely over the brain. It follows from these two premises that certain lesions, the gross symptoms of which do not differ materially, must still differ in their psychological effects

(Freud, 1953[1891], p. 17)

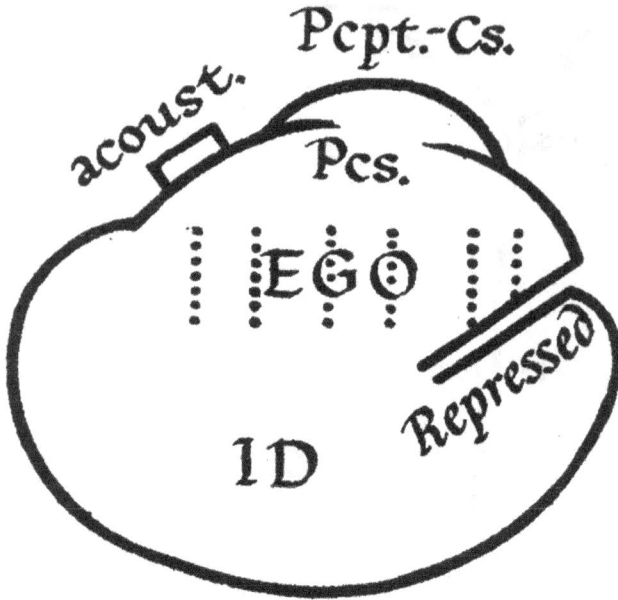

Figure 2.22 Freud's diagram representing 'the spatial or "topographical" idea of mental life'.

This illustrates Freud's interest in exploring an integrated theory of the brain (and shows building blocks to his psychoanalytic theory which will come later), in spatial versus integrated, he is writing that integrated thinking and functioning is still spatial, but not in the form of localized functions previously accepted by neurologists. Integration integrates is the way forward in theoretical terms. Throughout his work, he developed theory on the integration of mind and body. This may give us a sense of why his own spatialising, and theory about spatialising was minimized, although place remains, as in the ego, id, super-ego, ego-ideal of the structural model. These locations are places, and the places are sets of agencies such as the internal world as Klein conceives of it. Wollheim writes about states of mind directed upon spatial things:

> It is clearly not enough, for a conception of the mind to be reckoned spatial, that we should attribute to the mind states which have as their objects, or are directed upon, things that are themselves spatial: for instance, the fact that we attribute to the mind thoughts about people and scenes, which are three-dimensional.
>
> (Wollheim, 1969, p. 216)

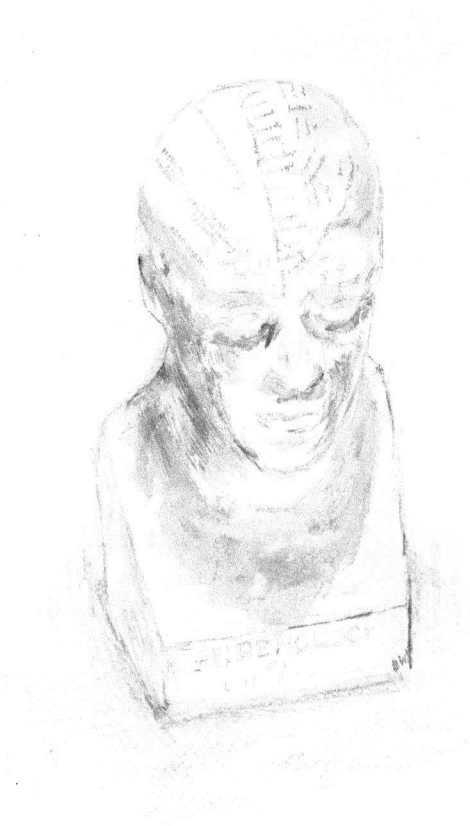

Figure 2.23 Drawing of a Phrenology head. Drawing by D. Wright.

and that the mind is 'a theatre upon whose stage the figures of fancy or imagination make their appearance. (Wollheim, 1969, p. 213) Wollheim writes about psychotic spatialising which is even more primitive:

> I should reckon it both proper and illuminating to say that our ordinary conception of the mind, while not that of a place, is one which, when distorted, is that of a place. This distortion, spelt out, is the story of our life read in reverse: as such, it marks the path of a regression. Now I may have suggested that the conception of mind involved in the unconscious states we have been considering in some detail is a fully spatial conception: which would be wrong. For there are conceptions that go beyond it in spatiality: conceptions, in other words, more distorted yet. I

now want to suggest that it might be possible to characterize the varying stages of mental disturbance, or the stations on the path to psychosis, by the degree to which the patient conceives of the mind, supremely of his mind, as a place.

(Wollheim, 1969, p. 217)

Wollheim is saying that the more one can think in one's own mind about one's mind, then spatialising is reduced; however, the extreme end of spatialising is psychosis. This is related to Freud's (1907) writing on obsessive thinking and actions and the chair in the consulting room (see p. X) being used for these purposes. This is what my study will take up where this has remained untheorized.

In this chapter, I looked at Freud's use of space and meaning of locality, spatial diagrams as well as projection of maternal and paternal figures into the space of rooms. I suggest the first spatialising of which Freud was consciously aware (matrix stage 2, *Room-object* may have been the 'cabinet' which was introjected and re-projected into many of Freud's rooms, including his own consulting room. I suggest that evidence of spatialisation into rooms by Freud has not been taken up in psychoanalytic theory, perhaps because it was so personal and habitual for Freud and perhaps not entirely conscious. Then later generations, in identification with Freud, repeat his retaining of spatialisation in an unconscious or minimally conscious state. That is why there is so little literature about it. However, Freud's fascination with the development of the mind included his attempt to find the original spatialisation, which creates the object world and is retained in transferences. Freud's conceptualization of projection (unformed internal pressure of instinct put into spatial form) is necessarily spatial and I utilise his instinct theory for building my alternative concept. Wollheim wrote that the more we look at the mind's primitive state the more we see spatialisation. I will go on in the following chapter 3 to look at the construction of my concept in view of what is missing in current theory and showing the current theory utilised to construct it.

Figure References

Figure 2.1: Sigmund Freud's diagrams of Mnemic symbols – S. Freud. Freud, S. (1953[1900]). The Interpretation of Dreams. Tr. & ed. James Strachey et al. Standard Edition of the Complete Psychological Works of Sigmund Freud, vol IV. London: Hogarth Press and the Institute of Psychoanalysis. (First Part), ix-627. (pages 538 & 541). **By permission of The Marsh Agency Ltd on behalf of Sigmund Freud Copyright.**

Figure 2.2: Map of Trieste, where Sigmund Freud's room in "Zoologische Station" was located by S. Freud, in: Freud, S. (1990 [1876]) Letter from

Sigmund Freud to Eduard Silberstein April 5, 1876. The Letters of Sigmund Freud to Eduard Silberstein 1871–1881, 142–150. Ed: Walter Boehlich. Cambridge, MA. Harvard University Press. (page 143). **By permission of The Marsh Agency Ltd on behalf of Sigmund Freud Copyright.**

Figure 2.3: Drawing of Sigmund Freud's room in "Zoologische Station" in Trieste by S. Freud, in: Freud, S. (1990 [1876]) Letter from Sigmund Freud to Eduard Silberstein April 5, 1876. The Letters of Sigmund Freud to Eduard Silberstein 1871–1881, 142–150. Ed: Walter Boehlich. Cambridge, MA. Harvard University Press. (page 143). **By permission of The Marsh Agency Ltd on behalf of Sigmund Freud Copyright.**

Figure 2.4: Page of Letter from Sigmund Freud to Eduard Silberstein April 5, 1876, showing Freud's diagrams of his Desk and Chair (Copy in the Special Collection of University of Essex Library). **With thanks to the University of Essex Library Staff. By permission of The Marsh Agency Ltd on behalf of Sigmund Freud Copyright.**

Figure 2.5: Drawing of Sigmund Freud's table in his room in "Zoologische Station" in Trieste by S. Freud, in: Freud, S. (1990 [1876]) Letter from Sigmund Freud to Eduard Silberstein April 5, 1876. The Letters of Sigmund Freud to Eduard Silberstein 1871–1881, 142–150. Ed: Walter Boehlich. Cambridge, MA. Harvard University Press. (page 143). **By permission of The Marsh Agency Ltd on behalf of Sigmund Freud Copyright.**

Figure 2.6: Drawing of Sigmund Freud's chair in his room in "Zoologische Station" in Trieste by S. Freud, in: Freud, S. (1990 [1876]) Letter from Sigmund Freud to Eduard Silberstein April 5, 1876. The Letters of Sigmund Freud to Eduard Silberstein 1871–1881, 142–150. Ed: Walter Boehlich. Cambridge, MA. Harvard University Press. (page 143). **By permission of The Marsh Agency Ltd on behalf of Sigmund Freud Copyright.**

Figure 2.7: Drawing of S. Freud's room in the "The General Hospital" in Vienna by S. Freud in letter to Martha Bernays, October, 1883. In Freud, E., Freud, L. & Grubrich-Simitis, I. (1978 [1998])) Sigmund Freud his life in pictures and words. London, W.W. Norton and Company Limited (page 150). **By permission of The Marsh Agency Ltd on behalf of Sigmund Freud Copyright.**

Figure 2.8: Drawing of an aerial of Freud's Room (by D. Wright) as described in Freud, S (1961 [1882]) Letter from Sigmund Freud to Martha Bernays, June 19, 1882. Letters of Sigmund Freud 1873–1939, 7–10. *Reproduced with permission of Palgrave Macmillan. from Wright, D. (2018) 'Rooms as Replacements for People: The Consulting Room as a Room*

Object' (pp. 251–262) in 'Psychoanalysis' section of 'On Replacement – Cultural, Social and Psychological Representations', Eds: Jean Owen and Naomi Segal, Switzerland, Palgrave Macmillan.

Figure 2.9: 'Little Hans is specially frightened when carts drive into or out of the yard' from Freud, S. (1955 [1909]). 'Analysis of a Phobia in a Five-Year-Old Boy'. Tr. & ed. James Strachey et al. Standard Edition of the Complete Psychological Works of Sigmund Freud, vol X. London: Hogarth Press and the Institute of Psychoanalysis. 1–150. (page 46). **By permission of The Marsh Agency Ltd on behalf of Sigmund Freud Copyright.**

Figure 2.10: Engraving by Eugene Pirodon of the oil painting by Pierre Aristide André Brouillet entitled 'A Clinical Lesson at the Salpêtrière' (1887) which hung in Sigmund Freud's consulting rooms in Berggasse 19 and Maresfield Gardens. **© Freud Museum London.**

Figure 2.11: Photograph by Edmund Engleman, 1938, showing engraving by Eugene Pirodon of the oil painting by Pierre Aristide André Brouillet entitled 'A Clinical Lesson at the Salpêtrière' (1887) hanging in Sigmund Freud's consulting rooms in Berggasse 19, on the top left hand side of the photograph **© Freud Museum London.**

Figure 2.12: Drawing of Maresfield Gardens showing engraving of the Charcot painting above the couch (top right). Drawing by D. Wright.

Figures 2.13: Photograph of Sigmund Freud's consulting room in Vienna, May 1938. Photograph by E Engleman. **© Freud Museum London.**

Figures 2.14: Photograph of Sigmund Freud's consulting room in Vienna, May 1938. Photograph by E Engleman. **© Freud Museum London.**

Figure 2.15: Sigmund Freud's room in Maresfield Gardens with his desk, chair and figures on the desk. Drawing by D. Wright.

Figure 2.16: Head in glass box in Sigmund Freud's study, Maresfield Gardens. Drawing by D. Wright.

Figure 2.17: Freud's drawing of the brain's workings (originally 'Figure 2. Schema 1/a and 1/b' p. 197), by S. Freud. Freud, S. (2012 [1887]) Critical Introduction to Neuropathology (1887). Psychoanalysis and History. 14(2):151–202. **By permission of The Marsh Agency Ltd on behalf of Sigmund Freud Copyright.**

Figure 2.18: Freud's drawing of the brain's workings (originally Figure 3. Schema 2: Tracts of the cerebral grey p. 198) by S. Freud. Freud, S. (2012 [1887]) Critical Introduction to Neuropathology (1887). Psychoanalysis and History. 14(2):151–202. **By permission of The Marsh Agency Ltd on behalf of Sigmund Freud Copyright.**

Figure 2.19: Freud's drawing of the brain's workings (originally Figure 4 Schema 3: Sensory nuclei and substantia reticularis p. 199) by S. Freud. Freud, S. (2012 [1887]) Critical Introduction to Neuropathology (1887). Psychoanalysis and History. 14(2):151–202. **By permission of The Marsh Agency Ltd on behalf of Sigmund Freud Copyright.**

Figure 2.20: Sigmund Freud's Fig 1 'Schematic Picture of Sexuality' [his Fig 1.] 'Schematic Picture of Sexuality' in Freud S. (1966 [1890]) Freud, S. (1966 [1892]). Draft G 1 Melancholia2 from Extracts From The Fliess Papers. Tr. & ed. James Strachey et al. Standard Edition of the Complete Psychological Works of Sigmund Freud, vol I. London: Hogarth Press and the Institute of Psychoanalysis. 200–206. (page 202). **By permission of The Marsh Agency Ltd on behalf of Sigmund Freud Copyright.**

Figure 2.21: Sigmund Freud's Fig 2 'Schematic Picture of Sexuality' [his Fig 2.] 'Schematic Picture of Sexuality' in Freud S. (1966 [1890]) Freud, S. (1966 [1892]). Draft G 1 Melancholia2 from Extracts From The Fliess Papers. Tr. & ed. James Strachey et al. Standard Edition of the Complete Psychological Works of Sigmund Freud, vol I. London: Hogarth Press and the Institute of Psychoanalysis. 200–206. (page 202). **By permission of The Marsh Agency Ltd on behalf of Sigmund Freud Copyright.**

Figure 2.22: Sigmund Freud's diagram representing 'the spatial or "topographical" idea of mental life in Freud, S. (1961 [1923]). The Ego and the Id. Tr. & ed. James Strachey et al. Standard Edition of the Complete Psychological Works of Sigmund Freud, vol XIX. London: Hogarth Press and the Institute of Psychoanalysis.1–66. **By permission of The Marsh Agency Ltd on behalf of Sigmund Freud Copyright.**

Figure 2.23: Drawing of a Phrenology head. Drawing by D. Wright.

References

Berke, J. H. (2015) *The Hidden Freud: His Hassidic Roots*. London: Karnac.
Doolittle, H. (2012 [1956]) *Tribute to Freud*. New York: New Directions Books.
Freud, E., Freud, L. & Grubrich-Simitis, I. (1998 [1978]) *Sigmund Freud his Life in Pictures and Words*. London: W.W. Norton and Company Limited.

Freud, S. (1940) An Outline of Psycho-Analysis. *International Journal of Psychoanalysis.* 21:27–84.

Freud, S. (1953 [1891] *On Aphasia A Critical Study*, Trans. And Intro E. Stengel, New York: International Universities Press.

Freud, S. (1953 [1890]) Psychical (or Mental) Treatment. Tr. & ed. James Strachey *et al. Standard Edition of the Complete Psychological Works of Sigmund Freud*, vol VII. London: Hogarth Press and the Institute of Psychoanalysis. 281–302.

Freud, S. (1953 [1900]) The Interpretation of Dreams. Tr. & ed. James Strachey *et al. Standard Edition of the Complete Psychological Works of Sigmund Freud*, vol IV. London: Hogarth Press and the Institute of Psychoanalysis. (First Part), ix–627.

Freud, S. (1953 [1905(1901)]) Fragment of an Analysis of a Case of Hysteria. Tr. & ed. James Strachey *et al. Standard Edition of the Complete Psychological Works of Sigmund Freud*, vol VII. London: Hogarth Press and the Institute of Psychoanalysis. 1–122.

Freud, S. (1955 [1909]) 'Analysis of a Phobia in a Five-Year-Old Boy'. Tr. & ed. James Strachey et al. *Standard Edition of the Complete Psychological Works of Sigmund Freud*, vol X. London: Hogarth Press and the Institute of Psychoanalysis. 1–150.

Freud, S. (1955 [1913]) Totem and Taboo. Tr. & ed. James Strachey *et al. Standard Edition of the Complete Psychological Works of Sigmund Freud*, vol XIII. London: Hogarth Press and the Institute of Psychoanalysis. vii–162.

Freud, S. (1955 [1923]) Two Encyclopaedia Articles. Tr. & ed. James Strachey *et al. Standard Edition of the Complete Psychological Works of Sigmund Freud*, vol XVIII. London: Hogarth Press and the Institute of Psychoanalysis. 233–260.

Freud, S. (1957 [1910]) Five Lectures on Psycho-analysis. Tr. & ed. James Strachey *et al. Standard Edition of the Complete Psychological Works of Sigmund Freud*, vol XI. London: Hogarth Press and the Institute of Psychoanalysis. 1–56.

Freud, S. (1957 [1915]) Instincts and their Vicissitudes. Tr. & ed. James Strachey *et al. Standard Edition of the Complete Psychological Works of Sigmund Freud*, vol XIV. London: Hogarth Press and the Institute of Psychoanalysis. 109–140.

Freud, S. (1958 [1913]) On Beginning the Treatment (Further Recommendations on the Technique of Psycho-Analysis I). Tr. & ed. James Strachey *et al. Standard Edition of the Complete Psychological Works of Sigmund Freud*, vol XII. London: Hogarth Press and the Institute of Psychoanalysis. 121–144.

Freud, S. (1959 [1907]) Obsessive Actions and Religious Practices. Tr. & ed. James Strachey *et al. Standard Edition of the Complete Psychological Works of Sigmund Freud*, vol IX. London: Hogarth Press and the Institute of Psychoanalysis. 115–128.

Freud, S. (1960 [1901]) The Psychopathology of Everyday Life. Tr. & ed. James Strachey *et al. Standard Edition of the Complete Psychological Works of Sigmund Freud*, vol VI. London: Hogarth Press and the Institute of Psychoanalysis. vii–296.

Freud, S. (1961 [1882]) Letter from Sigmund Freud to Martha Bernays, June 19, 1882. *The Letters of Sigmund Freud 1873–1939*, 7–10. Ed: Ernst Freud. Tr: Tania and James Stern. London: Hogarth Press.

Freud, S. (1961 [1882]) Letter to Martha Bernays, August 18, 1882. *The Letters of Sigmund Freud 1873–1939*, 25–28. Ed: Ernst Freud. Tr: Tania and James Stern. London: Hogarth Press.

Freud, S. (1961 [1883]) Letter from Sigmund Freud to Martha Bernays, October 9, 1883. *The Letters of Sigmund Freud 1873–1939*, 67–68. Ed: Ernst Freud. Tr: Tania and James Stern. London: Hogarth Press.

Freud, S. (1961 [1885]) Letter from Sigmund Freud to Martha Bernays, November 24, 1885. *The Letters of Sigmund Freud 1873–1939*, 184–187. Ed: Ernst Freud. Tr: Tania and James Stern. London: Hogarth Press.

Freud, S. (1961 [1923]) The Ego and the Id. Tr. & ed. James Strachey *et al. Standard Edition of the Complete Psychological Works of Sigmund Freud*, vol XIX. London: Hogarth Press and the Institute of Psychoanalysis. 1–66.

Freud, S. (1961 [1930]) Civilisation and its Discontents. Tr. & ed. James Strachey *et al. Standard Edition of the Complete Psychological Works of Sigmund Freud*, vol XXI. London: Hogarth Press and the Institute of Psychoanalysis. 57–146.

Freud, S. (1963 [1917]) Introductory Lectures on Psycho-Analysis. Tr. & ed. James Strachey *et al. Standard Edition of the Complete Psychological Works of Sigmund Freud*, vol XVI. London: Hogarth Press and the Institute of Psychoanalysis. (Part III), 241–463.

Freud, S. (1963 [1916]) Introductory Lectures on Psycho-Analysis. Tr. & ed. James Strachey *et al. Standard Edition of the Complete Psychological Works of Sigmund Freud*, vol XV. London: Hogarth Press and the Institute of Psychoanalysis. (Part I&II) 1–240.

Freud, S. (1964 [1936]) A Disturbance of Memory on the Acropolis. Tr. & ed. James Strachey *et al. Standard Edition of the Complete Psychological Works of Sigmund Freud*, vol XXII. London: Hogarth Press and the Institute of Psychoanalysis. 237–248.

Freud, S. (1966 [1892]) Draft G 1 Melancholia2 from Extracts From The Fliess Papers.Tr. & ed. James Strachey *et al. Standard Edition of the Complete Psychological Works of Sigmund Freud*, vol I. London: Hogarth Press and the Institute of Psychoanalysis. 200–206.

Freud, S. (1990 [1876]) Letter from Sigmund Freud to Eduard Silberstein April 5, 1876. *The Letters of Sigmund Freud to Eduard Silberstein 1871–1881*, 142–150. Ed: Walter Boehlich. Cambridge MA: Harvard University Press.

Freud, S. (2012 [1887]) Critical Introduction to Neuropathology (1887). *Psychoanalysis and History.* 14(2):151–202.

Gardiner, M. Ed. (1989 [1972]) Pankejeff, S. (Pseudonym The Wolf-Man) My Recollections of Sigmund Freud. Tr. Muriel Gardiner. In *The Wolf-Man and Sigmund Freud*. London: Karnac Books.

Gerald, M. (2009) In The Shadow of Freud's Couch: Portraits of Psychoanalysts in Their Offices. [Online]. (Accessed 3rd March 2015). Available from http://www.markgeraldphoto.com

Jones, E. (1967 [1953]) *The Life and Work of Sigmund Freud*. Harmondsworth: Penguin.

Mahon, E. (2005) Dreams of Architecture and the Architecture of Dreams. *Annual of Psychoanalysis*, 33:25–37.

Myers, W. A. (1994) Addictive Sexual Behavior. *Journal of the American Psychoanalytic Association.* 42:1159–1182.

Spankie, R. (2015) *Sigmund Freud's Desk An Anecdoted Guide*. London: Freud Museum London.

Walter, E. V. (1988) *Placeways: A Theory of the Human Environment*. Chappell Hill and London: UNC Press Books.

Werner, A. (2002) Edmund Engelman: Photographer of Sigmund Freud's Home and Offices. *International Journal of Psycho-Analysis*, 83(2):445–451.

Wollheim, R. (1969) The Mind and the Mind's Image of Itself. *International Journal of Psycho-Analysis*, 50:209–220.

Wright, D. (2018) Rooms as Replacements for People: The Consulting Room as a Room Object (pp. 251–262). In: *On Replacement – Cultural, Social and Psychological Representations*. Editors: Owen, J. and Segal, N., Switzerland: Palgrave Macmillan

Chapter 3

Spatial Concepts and Formulation of the Room-object Spatial Matrix

[This chapter contains material from

the book Chapter; Wright, D. (2018) 'Rooms as Replacements for People: The Consulting Room as a Room Object' (pp. 251–262) in 'Psychoanalysis' section of 'On Replacement – Cultural, Social and Psychological Representations', Eds: Jean Owen and Naomi Segal, Switzerland, Palgrave Macmillan.

And; Wright, D. (2019) 'Spatialisation and the Fomenting of Political Violence'(pp. 167–187) in Fomenting Political Violence – Fantasy, Language, Media, Action.', Eds. Steffen Kruger, Karl Figlio, Barry Richards. Switzerland, Palgrave Macmillan. Reproduced with permission of Palgrave Macmillan.]

In the previous chapter, I looked at spatialisation in Freud's writing. In this chapter, I use this as well as the historical, cultural, and anthropological material in Chapter 1 and the theory I discuss here of Object-Relational and Winnicottian theory, including the areas of incompleteness and my specific response to it, to construct my theoretical model formulation of the Room-object Spatial matrix.

Melanie Klein – Positions, the Spatial Aspects of Transference and the Inside of Mother's Body

Melanie Klein (1946) shows children's phantasies about what goes on inside mother's body as well as schizoid mechanisms, writing the following about what I see as a core dimension of spatialisation:

> The processes of splitting off parts of the self and projecting them into objects are [...] of vital importance for normal development as well as for abnormal object relations. [...] [W]hen the ego ideal is projected into another person, this object becomes predominantly loved and admired

DOI: 10.4324/9781003188117-3

because it contains the good parts of the self. Similarly, the relation to other persons on the basis of projecting bad parts of the self into them is of a narcissistic nature because in this case as well the object strongly represents one part of the self. [...] The need to control others can to some extent be explained by a deflected drive to control parts of the self. When these parts have been projected excessively into another person, they can only be controlled by controlling the other person.

(Klein, 1946, pp. 103–104)

In the case of the defence mechanism Klein describes above, I extend Klein's theory here, as the 'control' that Klein writes of, of bad, intolerable, anxiety-provoking feelings and thoughts, which cannot be contained in the self, does not only take place – or better: is not only placed within people, but rather within anything in the environment, such as buildings, rooms, and objects. This can be a notion of a room as a good mother, inside of which all is good and outside of which all is bad. Historically, I argue, this can be seen to relate to the splitting of the sacred and the profane. The primitive mechanism of spitting good and bad is utilised as part of the spatialisation process. The phenomena that I looked at in chapter 1, in the Nigerian village and Abbey examples of spatialisation, involve the splitting of sacred and profane which Klein writes of. In projective identification (1946) Klein suggests the projection is identified with by the receiver of the projection which increases the efficacy of the projection. In the case of spatialisation into room spaces, if the space is manipulated and modified to receive the projection and there is an unconscious phantasy, that the space will then effectively receive the projections, then this increases the efficacy of the successful projection of the feelings/instincts.

Klein's 'Paranoid Schizoid position' (1946) and the 'Depressive position' (1946) are oscillated in and out of depending on the capacity, need, and circumstances to tolerate internal object pressure. I build on this idea where my Room-object Spatialisation Matrix stages are moved in and out depending on need. Although spatialisation can be seen as a primitive mechanism utilised from birth as a part of emotional and psychological functioning, it is also frequently utilised in adulthood to retreat into – a defence to which the psyche retreats when stressed – as the mastery of the undifferentiated, relentless, internal pressure of instinct.

Donald Meltzer writes about the 'life-space' of organisms with a 'mental life' where this 'life-space may be said to comprise the various compartments of the *'geography of phantasy'* (Meltzer) moving on the dimension of time. This geography is ordinarily organized into four compartments: inside the self; outside the self; inside internal objects; inside external objects; and to these may sometimes, perhaps always, be added the fifth compartment, the 'nowhere' of the delusional system, outside the gravitational pull of good objects.' (Meltzer, 1975, p. 223; emphasis mine). Like Klein, Meltzer is writing about dimensions within and around the individual, in relation to introjection and projection (including projective identification), although his formulations are not explicitly related to what I call spatialising he is concerned with the *'geography of phantasy'*.

For Klein, transference has an essential spatial dimension, and in the consulting room an account of transference is not adequate without it. Hinshelwood wrote that:

> Klein laid down that the total of all free associations that come into a patient's mind can be referred to the transference, however remote from consciousness the link may be: 'For many years transference was understood in terms of direct references to the analyst in the patient's material. My conception of transference as rooted in the earliest stages of development and in deep layers of the unconscious is much wider and entails a technique by which from the whole material presented the *unconscious elements* of the transference are deduced'. (Klein, 1952, p. 55). This has developed as an emphasis on the total situation.
>
> (Hinshelwood, 1994[1989], p. 17)

I am adding to this theory by suggesting that there is a projection or rather re-projection to the consulting room that is related to previous projections onto rooms that were utilised for Room-object spatialisation. This re-projection may run parallel to a transference, but in addition may also be instead of it, as a separate pre-object, pre-transferential projection as well as a projection of the spatial aspect of mother, as seen in my hypothesised Matrix stage 3 *Secondary Spatialised Room-object in the Consulting Room.* I am not dismissing the idea of transference but there is a more elemental level – I am going to magnify that primitive spatial level of thinking.

Wilfred Bion and Containment

Wilfred Bion described his concept of containing, as a way of managing the threat of disintegration and what he would call 'nameless dread', (Bion, 1962, p. 309):

> When the patient strove to rid himself of fears of death which were felt to be too powerful for his personality to contain he split off his fears and put them into me, the idea apparently being that if they were allowed to repose there long enough they would undergo modification by my psyche and could then be safely reintrojected.
>
> (Bion, 1959, p. 312)

The mother, I suggest, is not only the first site of containment as Bion described it but also of the aspect of being an object that I have called spatialising. If the mother functions as a sufficiently good first object for the child's spatialising work, then part of the mother's role must be found in the process of containment (Bion, 1959), which involves the mother's mind being an auxiliary mind for that of the child. The mother detoxifies the raw emotions and thoughts by digesting them and feeding them back to the child in processed form. Through this process, the child learns how to think. I argue that, if the mother's capacity for this is insufficient, children begin to mark out spaces in their inanimate environment (such as rooms) as re-placements for the containing function. Thus, the mother is not only a spatialised object, but the non-containing mother forces the infant back on its earlier spatialisation, when it was first creating an object world. Mother, partly through being an object with objects inside, that is a projective target for the infant's earliest spatialisation, is then the source of transference, was also spatialised and so transference from her now included this spatialised aspect. Regressive reliance on spatialisation in the absence of maternal containment includes mother who is herself spatialised, which would then provide the spatialisation – invested in mother – to which the infant could then resort when other aspects of mother were lost. I am suggesting that adding to Bion's formulation of containment (Bion, 1959), if the mother is unavailable/partially unavailable to function as the container, then one option for the child is to create a rudimentary container for rudimentary detoxification via spatialisation (projection). Figlio and Richards (2003) specify the scope and nature of the containing function of nonhuman environments:

> this containing function, which I am attributing to street lighting, tarmac, and its postmodern equivalents, is not of the same order as the containing function of the mother or of any human agent. In a narrow, technical sense, what I am talking about is probably not containment because the container is not capable of receiving, responding to, and modifying the subject's projections [...]. There is projection, but no reception and detoxification as specified in Bion's concept of containment. [...] The role of the public utilities in the life of the mind must therefore be in an important way the creation *of* that mind, that is to say, their containing function must have been projectively invested in them.
>
> (Figlio & Richards, 2003, p. 412)

It is the projective investment, I argue, that is also the core driving force of the mechanism of spatialisation of projections; namely, to create a fantasy of containment. Fig. 3.1 shows a drawing of mine that illustrates the spatial array of rooms utilised through spatialisation to create some sort of containment through creating this rudimentary auxiliary mind which then can be introjected (taken inside) the mind. The meaning given to a space as a

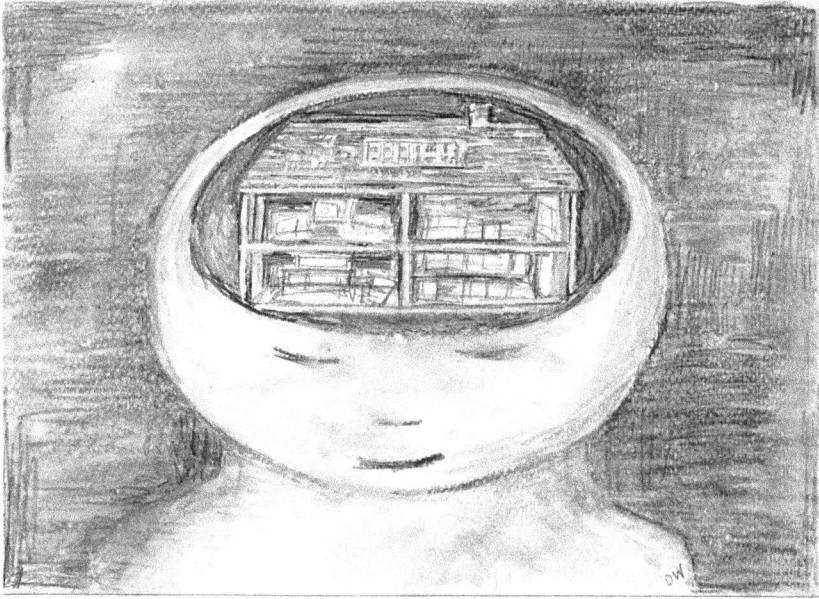

Figure 3.1 The Spatial Array of Rooms as an Auxiliary Mind. Drawing by D. Wright.

rudimentary mind, replaces the function of the mind of the mother and is then taken back inside the self (introjected), to act as an auxiliary thinking space. This rudimentary, auxiliary mind thus replaces a genuine capacity to think, with ideas that can be made to stand in for thinking (e.g., in the case of Fig. 3.1: rooms). I argue that this is precisely the objective of the mechanism of the spatialisation of projections; to create a fantasy containment. As I show in the case of the abbey, the containment happens through phantasy of the roll of the environment, it being the fantasy object to be controlled. If there has been insufficient containment in the early stages of development, then this may be the only kind of containment obtainable with a fantasised exchange like mother. So, transference from mother to a space, then the use of that space on its own as a resort when containment fails, becomes a replacement for mother and the space of mother's body and the space and containing function of her mind. This is perhaps what Bion wrote about in relation to the patient's relationships with rooms:

Presenter: **She told me since her mother's death she has kept her parent's bedroom intact; she has never moved any clothes, furniture, ornaments, or photographs.**
Bion: **The advantage of 'the facts' is that they make it easier to talk about the furniture of the room than the furniture of her mind or**

character. But it is a step in that direction; it is a way of 'getting to know' who she is. It is a sort of 'transient' relationship; a sort of 'transference'. It is felt to be more bearable to know your self than to be ignorant of your self. But on the way to knowing her self it is easier for this patient to know the furniture of her house. She might get to know the furniture of her mind in time. (Bion, 1994, Kindle location 2524)

I am going on to suggest that patients' relationship with the consulting room as a secondary spatialisation of their primary room spatialisation serves as a top-up to the containing, thinking, function of the therapist, just as the primary room spatialisation was a top-up to the mother function. And further patients who are unable to utilise the therapist in the transference, may need the consulting room to be in this top-up role, for them to engage in the therapeutic process at all.

Robert Young looks at various aspects of spatiality in psychoanalytic theory, such as containment, projective identification, potential space, transitional phenomena, countertransference and the analytic space. He wrote that '[t]he history of thought about the mind and feelings is a terrible muddle. What I am seeking is a sense of the possibility of mental space, not what's in it. The goal of humanity and of psychoanalysis is the facilitation of a suitable space for containing, ruminating and making use of experience (Young, 1994, p. 34).

Young is interested in space as a rich concept, a metaphor, rather than the literal idea of space as dimension, at a primitive or psychotic level, as Wollheim and Meltzer do and which I am developing in this study.

Donald Winnicott: Developmental Aspects of Theory, the Environmental Mother, the Intermediate Area, and the True Self

Donald Winnicott's theoretical stages or experiences relate to maturational achievements or processes which, all being well with the environmental conditions, are along a progressive trajectory. These include 'holding' (Winnicott, 2002[1967], p. 111), the 'mirror-role'(Winnicott, 2002[1967], p. 111), 'transitional objects' (Winnicott, 2002[1953], p. 1), 'intermediate area' (Winnicott 2002[1953], p. 14) and 'the capacity to be alone' (Winnicott, 1958, p. 416). For Winnicott, maturation entails the ability to lead a creative, individual, and meaningful life. When things go wrong in this maturational process, when mother is not 'good enough', and the baby is left waiting 'x + y + z' (Winnicott 2002[1967], p. 97), Winnicott suggests options such as the possibility of forming a 'True and false self' (Winnicott, 1965, p. 140) or the 'antisocial tendency' (Winnicott, 1975, p. 306). These are to defend against disintegration or annihilation of the self. Both of these options contain a 'hope' (Winnicott, 1975, p. 309) that the true self is still intact and protected and that creativity through the maturational processes can still be achieved. Winnicott wrote:

> As I have already indicated, one has to allow for the possibility that there cannot be a complete destruction of a human individual's capacity for creative living and that, even in the most extreme case of compliance and the establishment of a false personality, hidden away somewhere there exists a secret life that is satisfactory because of its being creative or original to that human being.
>
> (Winnicott, 2002[1971], p. 68)

However, Winnicott's trajectory is deficient. It is not just a question of whether everyone can manage, all or some of the time, to utilise the true and false self-positioning. Winnicott's theory of maturation lacks an essential component: Spatialisation. While his theories of psychic development address the task of adapting to an external world, none of them include the crucial fact that the external world is framed in spaces. I aim to make my point by comparing his theories with spatialisation. Spatialisation and its consequences, such as the stages of my hypothetical Room-object Spatialisation Matrix, clarify or extend object-relational thinking. In my view, transitional space implies a dimensional aspect, which is not explored. Spatialisation is the foundation of mental functioning and a site into which people retreat to gain stability, before moving again to a more symbolic level. As I have argued, spatialising starts with mother to spatialise into, but if mother is not good, spatialising 'tops up' the mother function in rooms. Following Winnicott, I am informed by his concept of a pre-object environmental mother which is projected onto the walls of the room in Room-spatialisation. This maintains 'hope' and defends against disintegrations, creating a 'holding' together mother substitute space, that allows for the self to feel intact.

W. Ronald D. Fairbairn – Splitting: Inside Bad and Outside Good

In William Ronald Fairbairn's theory, relating to the circumstances of deprivation discussed above, when mother is not 'good enough', good and bad objects are split. Splitting for Fairbairn is like that for Klein, but the 'good' is projected outside into mother and 'bad' inside to retain hope of things becoming better. Fairbairn wrote:

> The child not only internalizes his bad objects because they force themselves upon him and he seeks to control them, but also, and above all, because he *needs* them. If a child's parents are bad objects, he cannot reject them, even if they do not force themselves upon him; for he

cannot do without them. Even if they neglect him, he cannot reject them; for, if they neglect him, his need for them is increased.

(Fairbairn, 1992[1952]), p. 67)

My hypothesis gives another option: If mother is unavailable for spatialising, then the room becomes the projected mother function and the control, which Fairbairn and Klein suggest, is of the room. My formulation is an extension of Fairbairn's theory, as the good is projected outside to the room space (stand in for mother function) but the self is expanded into, merged with the room space enabling it, therefore, to also remains good.

Francis Tustin and Hard, Shell-like Encapsulation

My hypothetical formulation of Room-spatialisation is similar to Francis Tustin's, in that it takes up an aspect of Tustin's hard, reassuring, autistic object: That it has dimensions. Objects exist in space as finite. Tustin writes of Autistic encapsulation:

A hard, shell-like encapsulation is the psychodynamic differential diagnostic feature uniquely specific to autistic children. As Kanner realized, such children do not distinguish between live people and inanimate objects; they treat them both in the same way – by pressing against a hard wall, or against the hard part of a person as an inanimate object.

(Tustin, 1990, p. 17)

As with the above discussion regarding Winnicott's theory, where I have added that transitional objects can be spread out in space, in dimensions, I also suggest this, with Tustin's autistic object. As can be seen in figures 38 and 40, in my hypothesised Room-object Spatialisation Matrix, in my illustration for Stage 2 – *Room-object*, the figure presses itself against the wall/wallpaper. The figure in that image was based on early accounts of Ms B, (see page 98) whose case I will treat in more detail in Chapter 5, when she talked about her relationship with her bedroom as a child, rubbing her cheeks against the wallpaper and the walls to comforting herself. She said that she was conscious it was a comfort, as she felt very lonely and isolated and was often put in her room by her mother which was experienced as deprivation. Ms B was aware of making the wall a replacement for mother, whereas Tustin's description of the 'shell-like encapsulation' as more like my matrix, Stage 1 – *Primal Spatialisation*, where the room is pre-object more like Winnicott's environmental mother, but the dimensional aspect. It's not just that the feeling of the wall was comforting, but that, as in the case of Tustin's autistic objects, it was felt to have limits in which she was contained.

Harold Searles and the Non-human World

Harold Searles writes specifically of the non-human world: 'It is my conviction that there is within the human individual a sense, whether at a conscious or unconscious level, of *relatedness to his nonhuman environment*, that this relatedness is one of the transcendentally important facts of humans living' (Searles 1987[1960], p. 6). And he also writes of 'a matter of regression to a primitive level of thinking, comparable with that found in children and in members of so-called primitive cultures, a level of thinking in which there is a *lack of differentiation between* the concrete and the metaphorical.' (Searles, 1962, p. 23) I extend Searles thinking by adding spatialisation. His thinking on our relationship with the non-human world as well as the relationship between 'the concrete and the metaphorical' within it, is key to the building of my hypothetical formulations of spatialising and Room-spatialising. Searles also wrote about his relationship to early spaces:

> My personal psychoanalysis, which concluded 7 years ago, further deepened my appreciation of the significance of the non-human environment. I shall never forget, to give but one example, the grief I felt upon realising that the very building in which I had grown up, which had been sold some years before, was now lost to me forever.
>
> (Searles, 1962, p. x)

I extend the idea he puts forward about his attachment to early room spaces by creating the hypothetical formulation of Room-spatialisation that addresses and extends it.

Christopher Bollas – Nesting Places for Our Imagination

Christopher Bollas also writes about the loss of a favourite childhood place:

> I have suffered the shock of losing this favoured place, and until I die it shall always be somewhere in mind. To lesser and greater extent, this is true of all of us, especially when we move house. To leave a home, even when the contents go with us, is to lose the nooks and crannies of parts of ourselves, nesting places for our imagination.
>
> (Bollas, 2009, p. 49)

Bollas suggests that favoured places from childhood relate to the imagination, with a suggestion that they are part of the mind. I extend this and say that the space of a room can be introjected and then be re-projected into another room space or the consulting room.

John Stilgoe writes: 'If the house is the first universe for its young children, the first cosmos, how does its space shape all subsequent knowledge of other space, of any larger cosmos? Is that house "a group of organic habits" or even something deeper, the shelter of the imagination itself?' (Stilgoe, 2014[1994]: viii). Like Bollas, Stilgoe writes about imagination, and Stilgoe suggests that the first house as a formative space. I extend this by suggesting that it stands in for the mother function. Bachelard writes:

> [I]f I were asked to name the chief benefit of the house, I should say: the house shelters daydreaming, the house protects the dreamer, the house allows one to dream in peace. [...] it is because our memories of former dwelling-places are relived as daydreams that these dwelling-places of the past remain in us for all time. Now my aim is clear: I must show that the house is one of the greatest powers of integration for the thoughts, memories and dreams of mankind.
>
> (Bachelard, 2014[1958], p. 28)

Bachelard suggests that this formative space can develop integration of thinking and is relived 'as daydreams'. Adding to this, I suggest that my hypothetical formulation of Room-object spatialising can replace the mother function by creating an auxiliary mind in the space of the room, which can then be introjected, and re-created as an auxiliary mind through re-projection into other room spaces and the consulting room. While a house might be a transferential experience from mother, it is the space itself that I emphasise. That is not just an important dimension of mother in the transference, but at more primal level, mother herself is created as an object through spatialising her.

Didier Anzieu's 'Skin-ego'

Didier Anzieu writes that when the child has a difficult experience of being with the mother from the beginning, the Skin-ego provides 'a containing and unifying wrapping around the Self' (Anzieu, 2016[1995], p. 105). When things are more problematic in development, then:

> It needs strengthening. [...] The double wrapping – its own plus that of its mother – is gleaming and ideal; it provides the narcissistic personality with the delusion of being invulnerable and immortal. In the psyche it is represented by the phenomenon of the "double wall".
>
> (Anzieu 2016[1995], p. 135)

I am suggesting that this 'double wrapping', this "double wall", is even more cemented and solidified by projecting the mother's part of the double skin onto the actual walls of rooms. Anzieu wrote of a case study of a boy called Juanito:

Juanito, who suffered from a congenital deformity, had had to undergo an operation soon after he was born. [...] The turning-point in Juanito's treatment was a session in which he tore off a huge strip of paper from the wall; the washable paper was pasted up for children to paint freely on and that piece was not yet marked. He cut the paper into small pieces, got undressed and asked his therapist to stick the pieces all over his body, [...] In this way Juanito repaired the flaws in his Skin-ego caused by the lack of tactile and auditory contacts and bodily handling by his mother and other carers which had been unavoidable during his hospital stay.

(Anzieu, 2016, pp. 70–71)

This case is similar to the situation which Ms B described (see page 74 & 98) of touching the walls of the room and hugging them so she can feel hugged by them. I am suggesting that this patient Anzieu writes of, is demonstrating a Room-object spatialisation re-projection into the space of the consulting room, behaving towards it as if it was this additional skin, relating to Anzieu's concept of 'double-wall' (Anzieu 2016, p. 135), enwrapping or enveloping to replace mother. I build on this, with my hypothesis that the whole room and the spatial array of objects in its contents can be employed for Room-spatialisation purposes.

Esther Bick and the Skin Functioning as a Boundary

Esther Bick and Anzieu show that there is an awareness of spatialisation, albeit undeveloped, in that both focus on the containing, outer layer of the being – skin: How it is dealt with and experienced. As Bick writes:

in its most primitive form the parts of the personality are felt to have no binding force amongst themselves and must therefore be held together [...] by the skin functioning as a boundary. But this internal function of containing the parts of the self is dependant initially on the introjection of an external object, experienced as capable of fulfilling this function. [...] Until the containing functions have been introjected, the concept of a space within the self cannot arise.

(Bick, 1968, p. 484)

As mentioned above I am suggesting that I extend the skin function to the wall function and also extend Bick's theory by suggesting that the walls provide an auxiliary containing function in absence of the 'concept of a space within the self' for thinking (as also discussed by Wollheim [1969]).

Henri Rey's the 'Brick Mother' and the Spatial Development of the Infant

Dr John Steiner wrote in the Foreword to Rey 1994 book 'Universals of psychoanalysis in the treatment of psychotic and borderline states' about Rey's use of the term 'brick mother' that he is famous in the psychoanalytic community for calling the Maudsley hospital where he worked for 'much of his professional life' (Steiner [in Rey], 1994, p. ix), but did not write about formally:

> Henri Rey has a special affection for the Maudsley, which he would refer to as 'the brick mother', and this is partly because of his gratitude to the shelter and opportunity it gave him early in his career. He saw how important the hospital was a safety for patients who were afraid of breaking down, and that it offered a kind of continuity and stability. He also recognized that this kind of 'brick mother' could be cold and unresponsive, but this was often compensated for by his personal warmth and enthusiasm. In this setting, Rey was always reminded of the terrible suffering experience by psychotic and borderline patients, and he remained distressed by patients for longer and in a deeper way than most of his hardened colleagues. [...] These patients have helped Rey to recognise the essentially spatial structure of the mind and to see how this evolved in relating to objects who are also represented spatially. The self may in this way be felt to reside in an object, and the process of differentiations requires a specific disengagement and emergence form the object. Rey writes in an original and enlightening way about such spatial relationships. For example, he describes how psychological birth need not correspond with biological birth since the infant often feels he retains so close a dependence on his mother that he lived in a kind of marsupial space, like the newborn kangaroo in his pouch, and true psychological birth requires a further process of separation, loss and mourning. A knowledge of these processes is essential for the understanding of phobic patients who feel they have discovered a safe haven and consider that they have been forced prematurely to emerge from the maternal space into a world for which they are not yet ready.
>
> (Steiner [in Rey], 1994, p. ix)

Rey makes and an important link for the patients of the building of the hospital being part of the treatment as the biding become a good mother object. This links to my exploration of a projection onto the space of the consulting room as separate to the therapist, although for Rey this is a transference onto the space rather than necessarily a transference from a previous building, although as he famously used this term in speech and did not develop it theoretically in my text it is difficult to say how he would have theoretically described this. Steiner goes on to describe Rey's formulation of 'spatial development' (Rey, 1994, p. 25) relating to mother (and Mother's body) in relation to safety and separation with the example of marsupial pouched. As Rey writes,

> 'We know that phobics avoid certain situations, for instance eating in public; they will not go to a restaurant, or to the cinema, or to shops. They restrict their outside space until they are housebound. It is important to understand what the ultimate space into which they retire corresponds to in the unconscious. The outside world or outside space is in such an instance transformed by projective identification into the body or internal space of the subject of him or herself, identified with the internal space of mother. This entering and coming out of a room is coming out of that which the room stand for- ultimately – the mother's body.
>
> (Rey, 1994, p. 25)

Again, for Rey, the space outside becomes a projection of the body or internal space of mother, rather than from a previous room space as a top up to the functioning of which I suggest could include the need for a 'spatial development' separate from mother through usage of room spaces to top of or fill in for closeness and/or safety with mother, so kangaroo pouch becomes the actual room. Rey's ideas on 'phobics' and safety is also relevant to thinking about a regressive potential that people may have taken up when being in or coming out of Covid-19 'lock down' and will be referred to in Chapter 6 in relation to that. I also refer to the 'brick mother' in Chapter 8 where I think about the Ending Room-object experience being in the hospital setting (see page 181).

The Stages of the Proposed Formulation of the Room-object Spatial Matrix Beginning With the Room-object Spatial Matrix Stage I – Primal Spatialisation

I will now set out what I call the Room-object Spatial Matrix in the five stages that constitute developmental but can be seen as a matrix of stages or 'positions;' can be moved in and out (or up and down through the Matrix).

The Room-object Spatialisation Matrix: *Stage 1 – Primal Spatialisation* is where parts of the mother's body are spatialised to constitute the object. It is the pre-object, pre-transferential creation of mother, where spatialising is a method of creating an object, bringing together parts of the object to form a whole, which is retained in transferences. This is what is new: It is developmentally prior to object relations and therefore to transference. The primitive target of the babies' earliest spatialisation and the source of future transference. It is the beginnings of anchoring experience in perceptual reality, which is spatial. It is the primitive establishment of objects by having dimensions, being in space. *Primal Spatialisation* underlies all spatialisation activity, so all spatialisation is like the original spatialisation of mother as an object from parts of mother/mother's body, and thus creating the object action is re-enacted via spatialisation to defend against the losing or damaging of the object the object.

Room-object Spatial Matrix: Stage 2 – Room-object

In Room-object Spatial Matrix *Stage 2 – Room-object* (see Fig. 3.2): I suggest that difficulty in utilising mother as the first object of spatialisation can lead to spatialising into the spatial array of room spaces to replace or supplement the mother function. This second stage is an introjection of the maternal object and a re-projection into a 'room', which can also be transferred to specific rooms. The room becomes a collection of objects as part of a whole mother with objects inside her or dispersed around her body from which the object is constructed. The room in which spatialisation

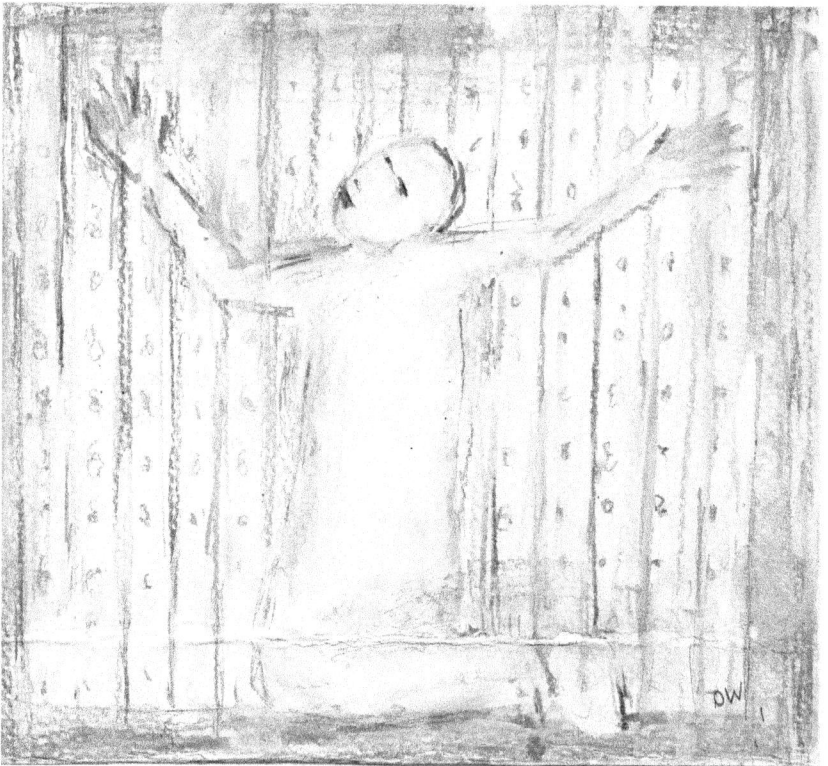

Figure 3.2 Room-object Spatial Matrix: Stage 2 – Room-object, which tops up the mother function. Painting by D. Wright.

occurs can be the means of anchoring experience in perceptual reality, which is spatial, as a stand in or top-up to the mother/object function. The room is a substitute mother/mother function. It is a transference from mother to a space, then that space is used, on its own, as a resort when containment fails, fulfilling the mother function as an auxiliary containing space. Spatialising into the spatial array of room spaces and the objects within them replaces or supplements the mother function, topping up the object usage of parts of mother including the insides and parts of the insides of mother, the outsides of mother and parts thereof, including mothers' skin, which can be spatialised in the outside and inside of the room walls and room contents. This *Room-object* gets used to make the room an object as a defensive reaction to maternal failure, a regressive defence and pathway to maturation. The primary room transference may have been re-spatialised multiple times before secondary spatialised in the consulting room.

Room-object Spatial Matrix Stage 3 – Consulting Room-object

The Room-object Spatial Matrix *Stage 3 – Consulting Room-object* (see Fig. 3.3) is where the consulting room is used as the original room was

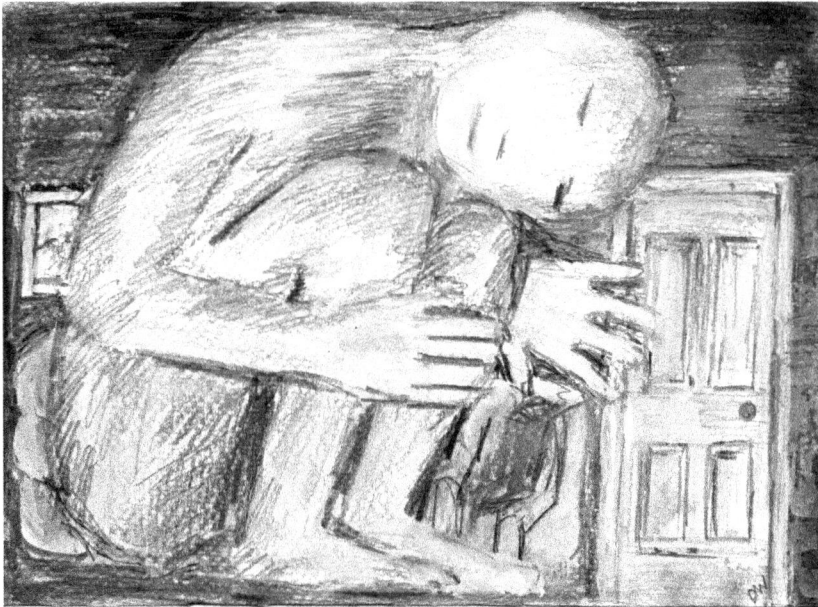

Figure 3.3 Room-object Spatial Matrix: Stage 3 – Consulting Room-object, in the Consulting Room. Painting by D. Wright.

used for *Stage 2 – Room-object,* as a direct displacement from one to another, separate from the transference to the therapist as an object. It is a relationship with the consulting room as a representative of the original primary spatialised room, this also includes the spatial array of spaces around the consulting room – such as the toilet, hallway, and so on and can be extended to the street. Just as in the Stage 2 – *Room-object* room, features of the Primary Spatialised Room stand out because they stand in for features of mother, here in this Stage 3 – *Consulting Room-object,* features of the consulting room also stand in for the features of mother as the *Room-object* did, and also the consulting room has features that stands in for the *Room-object* itself. In addition, the original *Room-object* may have been re-spatialised multiple times into other rooms before the consulting room, so therefore features of the consulting room may stand in for those other re-spatialised rooms also. In the case of Stage 3, this can happen before the patient is able to utilise the therapist very much at all, or able to relate to the therapist transferential, therefore the role of the consulting room is providing a very important function as enabling the patient to engage.

Room-object Spatial Matrix Stage 4 – Consulting Room-object + Transference

In the Room-object Spatial Matrix *Stage 4 – Consulting Room-object + transference* (see Fig. 3.4) secondary spatialisation occurs in exactly the same way as Stage 3 – *Consulting Room-object* (described above), except here in Stage 4, the spatialisation also includes the transference to the therapist as the object. Therefore, aspects of the Consulting Room, as the object/therapist's room, are also associated with the therapist as object constituents of the object therapist, so for example a cushion could represent part of the therapist's body/skin.

Room-object Spatial Matrix Stage 5 – Consulting Room-object + Transference Outside the Consulting Room

The Room-object Spatialisation Matrix, Stage 5 – *Consulting Room-object + Transference outside the Consulting Room* stage specifically refers to what goes on back outside the consulting room (outside the session) after being in or whilst in the consulting room (Fig. 3.5). It is a re- spatialisation of the consulting room outside the room. So, this includes the original *Stage 2 Room-object* of mother/object transference to the original room and all re-spatialised rooms before the consulting room (Fig. 3.2). It also includes *Stages 3 – Consulting Room*-object and *Stage 4 Consulting Room-object + transference.* This *Stage 5 – Consulting Room-object + Transference outside the Consulting Room* can function as a top-up to the function and role of the

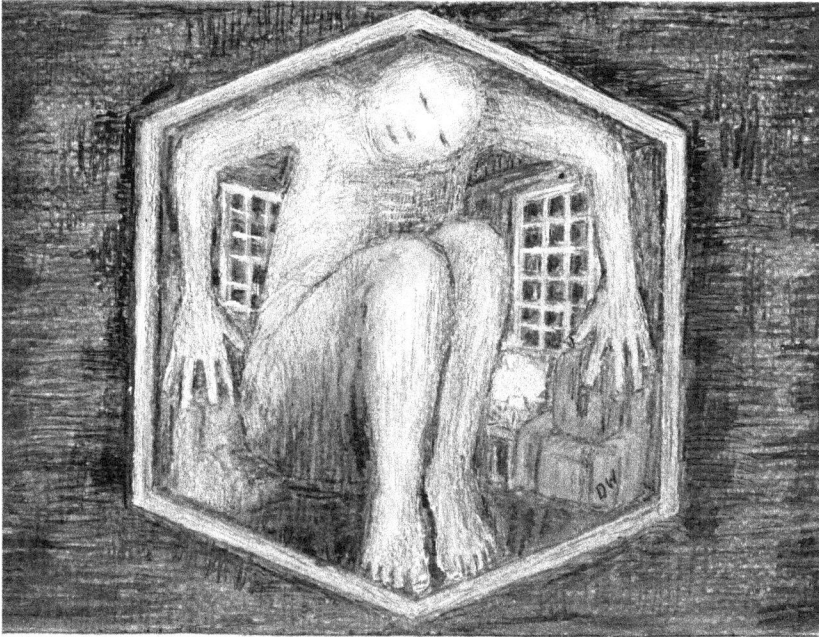

Figure 3.4 Room-object Spatial Matrix: Stage 4 – Consulting Room-object + Transference. Drawing by D. Wright.

consulting room as a container as separate from and alongside the therapist as the object in the transference.

The Role of the Consulting Room, Dimensions, Space, and Architecture in Psychoanalysis

Now that my alternative formulations of the Room-object spatial Matrix have been constructed, in the final section of this chapter, I will look at contemporary psychoanalytic thinking on the Role of the Consulting Room, dimensions, space, and architecture in Psychoanalysis to show where my formulation of the Room-object Spatial Matrix adds to current thinking on the space of the Consulting room.

As referred to in Chapter 2 (see page 51), Myers wrote of the use of a rug in the consulting room. He writes that after giving an interpretation to his patient, 'she began to rock back and forth and to cry. She took one of the Moroccan carpets I have thrown across my couch and wrapped herself in it, as in a swaddling blanket. The transformation from seductress one moment to wounded child the next was quite startling (Myers, 1994, p. 1167). The object in the room (carpet) appears to have had a transformative role in the

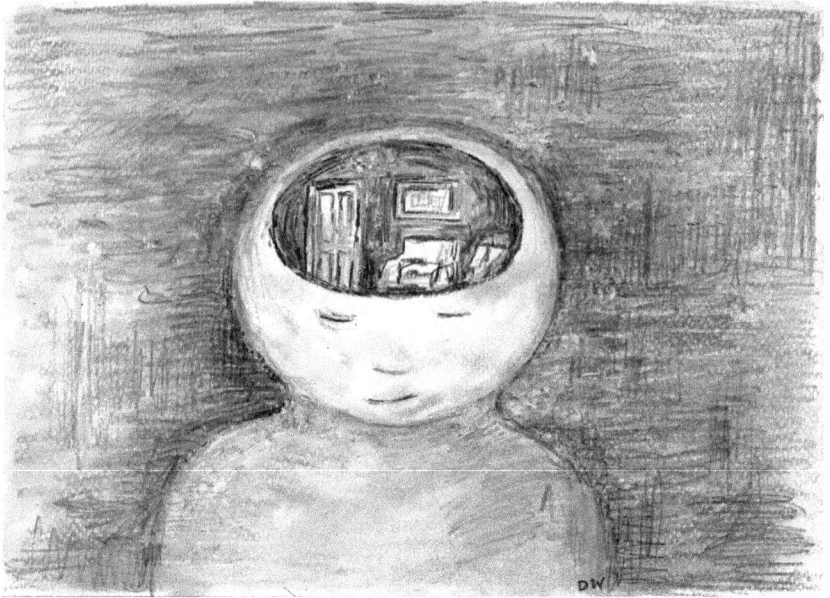

Figure 3.5 Room-object Spatial Matrix: Stage 5: Consulting Room-object + Transference, outside the Consulting room. Drawing by D. Wright.

work alongside the interpretation. This is what I am calling spatialisation, though in this Myers's case, as discussed in Chapter 2, I suggest that there is an almost third-hand spatialisation – the first spatialisation of the carpets being Freud in his own consulting room – the first consulting room, the second by Myers who found it meaningful to have the rugs in relation to Freud's consulting room, and third the patient who was able to utilise it the rug in a spatialised way, we could say in relation to the Matrix in a *Stage 4 Consulting Room-object + Transference*.

Michael Parsons wrote of the space of the consulting room that, '[t]he internal analytic setting is a psychic arena in which reality is defined by such concepts as symbolism, fantasy, transference, and unconscious meaning. These operate throughout the mind, of course. [...] Just as the external setting defines and protects a *spatiotemporal* arena in which patient and analyst can conduct the work of analysis (Parsons, 2007, p. 1444; emphasis mine). Michael Parsons suggests that in the 'spatiotemporal arena' of the consulting room, symbolism, fantasy, and transference are present, by which he infers that symbolism and fantasy might be additional to transference, but he does not go further into this idea in relation to the role of the consulting room, or look at a parallel transference to the room. Stephen Kurtz writes of the consulting room as a 'shared space – jointly created by analyst and patient – belonging to the realms of play and theatre. [...] [A] new playground in the safety of the consulting room.' (Kurtz, 1986, pp. 100–102), which suggests relating and transference and Patrick Casement refers to 'relationship-space' (Casement, 1999[1985], p. 192). We should note that 'space' is commonly used in psychoanalytic writing but without regard to its essential physical spatial reference. Elizabeth Danze wrote about the consulting room from an architectural perspective, where '[t]his special room becomes the explicit and specific territory of this uniquely formed relationship. There is no other *architectural space* that has precisely the same programmatic demands as this one. [...] At the same time, the objects, items, and art present in the room might provide opportunities for the association. (Danze, 2005, pp. 109–118; emphasis mine). Elizabeth Danze considers the 'specialness' of the physical space of the consulting room, with some descriptive architectural language and an idea of the importance of the space and the contents. She provides no case study, however, and therefore does not exemplify the possible meaning for a patient of this architectural space.

Henry Abramovitch takes up the case of moving consulting rooms, which I will explore in detail in the next Chapter 4, as well as Chapter 5 and Chapter 6 where I consider the Virtual Room move. He points out that, 'the move was a case of 'temenos lost' [...] at the time of a move, a dialectic between 'therapeutic relationship' and 'therapeutic space' emerges. A move disrupts the therapeutic unity of 'person-place' and forces the participants to confront how much of the therapeutic process is dependent upon the transference to *place* (Abramovitch, 1997, pp. 570–572; emphasis mine). This is important as consulting room moves are rarely referred to in literature, in relation to the patient's experience of them. This is also important as he has identified a 'transference to place'. He suggests its importance, but does not explicitly say that it is separate from transference to the therapist. However, in referring to the room as the 'Temenos' (a sacred space in a Greek temple precinct), he is thinking about the room itself having a healing entity of its own and opportunity for transference. His use of 'Temenos' is much like Freud's description of the 'purificatory baths, or the elicitation of oracular dreams by sleeping in the temple precincts, can only have had a curative effect by psychical means' (Freud, 1953[1890], p. 292). Sylvia O'Neill writes about the crea-tivity in the consulting room being facilitated by 'Donnet's theory of the analytic site' of the consulting room. She discusses this with a case study; 'Carl asked whether, during his sessions, it would be possible for the wall clock to be removed, or moved at least from his visual field. In a previous psychotherapy the loudly ticking desk clock, which had disturbed him, had been obligingly shut away by the therapist in the desk. [...] I told Carl that [...] perhaps in the course of his treatment we might be able to enquire into, and possibly come to understand, what was so disturbing for him about it. [...] the factor that facilitates creativity is the setting, or *site*, and the patient's transformational introjection of it. (O'Neill, 2015, pp. 466–474; emphasis mine) Like Abramovitch, O'Neill suggests that the Consulting room has an innate healing possibility which is less about projecting, more archetypal, but nevertheless points to a possible usage of the space as well as the therapist which again, we could think of as *Stage 5 – Consulting Room-object + Transference*.

Marilyn Mathew writes about a female patient's experience outside the consulting room, in her own bedroom, in which she, 'seems to have latched on through the window to the wind in the tree tops – [...] perhaps an unconscious reminder of the paintings of trees in my consulting room. By anchoring her external vision she found that she could let go and open up enough to allow the process of reverie and re-integration to spin a stronger internal structure and a more flexible containing membrane around herself' (Mathew, 2005, p. 387). The visual memory of the painting seemed to act as an important mechanism for linking the two rooms, the room at home and the consulting room, although the actual painting is not described in the paper. Here is a reference to an item from the consulting room that has been effectively (in my formulation) introjected and then re-projected to the view out of the window of the room. This seems to suggest an efficaciousness of the experience at home relating to the consulting room introjected. This could be thought of as a Matrix Stage 5 Consulting Room-object + Transference, outside the Consulting room. Benjamin Brent also provides a case study in which the physicality of the room is prominent in the work; 'It was the first day of our psychotherapy. James walked into my office and before I had the opportunity to recommend a place to sit, he said, "That's my chair," and sat down. [...] Of the two chairs, one—the one in which James seated himself—was situated at the desk. My briefcase rested just next to it. I sat down in the unoccupied chair and began to wonder what this meant [...]. Over the next several weeks, James and I engaged in a sort of musical chairs. (Brent, 2009, pp. 809–810). As it continues Brent gives interpretations and thoughts to the patient regarding the meaning of what is happening in the space. Although Brent's case study is brief, it is a good illustration of the importance of the physicality of the room within the psychoanalytic work, considering the importance of the objects in the room as they are seen and used symbolically and become of therapeutic importance (as they can be used for spatialisation in the spatial array of the consulting room). This is reminiscent of Freud's (1907) paper on the meaning of the chair in the room (as discussed on p. 50). One could argue that it is a straight transference, with the patient putting the analyst in place of the father, and expropriating his dominance, however, the mechanism is nonetheless spatial.

Rosine Jozef Perelberg looks at space in relation to time, phantasy, and memory; 'Within the analytic space, different dimensions of time unfold, and a tension between the old and the new is set in motion, In between the patient's presentation [...] and the analyst's response through his internal work [...] specific dimensions of time and space are created in the context of that relationship (Perelberg, 2008, p. 132), and that there are patients who fill the consulting room not only with their emotions and their actions, but also with their words, dreams, and associations (Perelberg, 2008, p. 870). Andrea Sabbadini also focusses on the time boundaries of the analytic space as well as the physical boundaries of the consulting room. It seems that 'space' needs to be differentiated, and it seems that my stages of spatialisation capture the possible range of meaning here. Cosimo Schinaia looks at different aspects of architecture from a psychoanalytic perspective, including the consulting room, but does not discuss theory relating to the role of the consulting room. Shannon Hendrix, and Lorens Eyan Holm, (2016) edit this book of the writings of architects (including Jane Rendell [below]) on 'Architecture and the Unconscious' using some psychoanalytic theory to describe and make sense of the architectural spaces. However, they also do not discuss theory relating to the role of the consulting room. Jane Rendell (2017) looks at architecture relating to Russian constructivist theory, where she uses some psychoanalytic theory, such as transitional space, as well as using diagrams by Freud, as illustrations, she offers no explanation at all about how they fit with her theories, and she draws very little from psychoanalytic thinking in relation to the architectural spaces she describes Something is getting recognised as important spatially but there is no current theory that explains this. The constructed theory in this chapter of the Room-object Spatial Matrix, informed by Psychoanalytic spatial theory (at the beginning of this chapter), Freud's Room-object spatialisation (Chapter 2) and historical and anthropological materials (Chapter 1) explain this further. Current psychoanalytic thinking on the consulting room was then examined, which does not usually distinguish spatialisation as a concrete phenomenon, from space as a metaphor for various ideas, such as containment and thinking itself, as in thinking space. This deficit makes the following study in Chapter 4 timely, which will show Clinical examples from the original study demonstrating my Room-object Spatial Matrix stages, with particular interest to the points at which the non-transferential stages occur in the material to see how and where it could be seen to inform and aid clinical understanding in practice of the patient's clinical material.

Figure References

Figure 3.1: The Spatial Array of Rooms as an Auxiliary Mind, Drawing by D. Wright. ***Reproduced with permission of Palgrave Macmillan*** *from Wright, D. (2019) 'Spatialisation and the Fomenting of Political Violence' in Fomenting Political Violence – Fantasy, Language, Media, Action.', Eds. Steffen Kruger, Karl Figlio, Barry Richards. Switzerland, Palgrave Macmillan. Reproduced with permission of Palgrave Macmillan.*

Figure 3.2: Room-object Spatial Matrix: Stage 2 – Room-object, which tops up the mother function. Painting by D. Wright.

Figure 3.3: Room-object Spatial Matrix: Stage 3 – Consulting Room-object, in the Consulting Room. Painting by D. Wright.

Figure 3.4: Room-object Spatial Matrix: Stage 4 – Consulting Room-object + Transference. Drawing by D. Wright.

Figure 3.5: Room-object Spatial Matrix: Stage 5 – Consulting Room-object + Transference, outside the Consulting room. Drawing by D. Wright.

References

Abram, J. and Hinshelwood, R. D. (2018) *The Clinical Paradigms of Melanie Klein and Donald Winnicott Comparisons and Dialogues*. Oxon: Routledge.

Abramovitch, H. (1997) Temenos lost: Reflections on moving. *Journal of Analytical Psychology*. 42(4), 569–584.

Anzieu, D. (2016) *The Skin-ego*. tr. Naomi Segal. London: Karnac.

Bachelard, G. (2014 [1958]) *The Poetics of Space*. tr. Maria Jolas. New York: Penguin Books.

Bick, E. (1968) The Experience of the Skin in Early Object – Relations. *The International Journal of Psycho-Analysis*. 49:484–486.

Bion, W. R. (1959) Attacks on Linking. *The International Journal of Psycho-Analysis*. 40:308–315.

Bion, W. R. (1962) The Psycho-Analytic Study of Thinking. *The International Journal of Psycho-Analysis*. 43:306–310.

Bion, W. R. (1994) *Clinical Seminars and Other Works*. London: Karnack Books.

Bollas, C. (2009) *The Evocative Object World*. East Sussex: Routledge.

Brent, B. (2009) Mentalization – Based Psychodynamic Psychotherapy for Psychosis. *Journal of Clinical Psychology: In Session*. 65(8):803–814. [Online]. [Accessed 29th March 2015]. Available from: http://singlecasearchive.com/node/2

Casement, P. (1999 [1985]) *On Learning From the Patient*. London: Routledge.

Danze, E. A. (2005) An Architect's View of Introspective Space The Analytic Vessel. Ann. Psychoanal. 33:109–124.

Fairbairn, W. D. (1992 [1952]) *Psychoanalytic Studies of the Personality*. London: Routledge.

Figlio, K., Richards, B. (2003) The Containing Matrix of the Social. *American Imago*. 60:407–428.

Freud, S. (1953 [1890]) Psychical (or Mental) Treatment. Tr. & ed. James Strachey *et al. Standard Edition of the Complete Psychological Works of Sigmund Freud*, vol VII. London: Hogarth Press and the Institute of Psychoanalysis. 281–302.

Freud, S. (1959 [1907]) Obsessive Actions and Religious Practices. Tr. & ed. James Strachey *et al. Standard Edition of the Complete Psychological Works of Sigmund Freud*, vol IX. London: Hogarth Press and the Institute of Psychoanalysis. 115–128.

Heimann, P. (1950) On Counter-Transference 1. *The International Journal of Psycho-Analysis.* 31:81–84.

Hendrix, J. S. and Holm, L. E. (Eds.) (2016) *Architecture and the Unconscious.* Dorchester: Dorset Press.

Hinshelwood, R. D. (1994 [1989]) *A Dictionary of Kleinian Thought.* London: Free Association Books.

Hinshelwood, R. D. (2013) *Research on the Couch Single-Case Studies, Subjectivity and Psychoanalytic Knowledge.* East Sussex: Routledge.

Klein, M. (1946) Notes on Some Schizoid Mechanisms. *The International Journal of Psycho-Analysis.* 27:99–110.

Klein, M. (1993 [1952]) Origins of Transference in The Writings of Melanie Klein, Vol. 3: Envy and Gratitude and Other Works 1946-1963, Karnac Books.

Kurtz, S. A. (1986) In the analytic theatre. Free Associations. 1(6):100–122.

Mathew, M. (2005) Reverie: Between thought and prayer. *Journal of Analytical Psychology,* 50(3):383–393.

Meltzer, D. (1975) Chapter IX: Dimensionality as a Parameter of Mental Functioning: Its Relation to Narcissistic Organisation. Explorations in Autism: *A Psycho-Analytical Study,* 223–238. Classic Books. Copyright 2018, Psychoanalytic Electronic Publishing. ISSN 2472-6982.

Myers, W. A. (1994) Addictive Sexual Behavior. *Journal of the American Psychoanalytic Association.* 42:1159–1182.

O'Neill, S. (2015) The Facilitating Function of the Setting. *British Journal of Psychotherapy.* 31(4):463–475.

Parsons, M. (2007) Raiding the Inarticulate: The Internal Analytic Setting and Listening Beyond Countertransference. *International Journal of Psycho-Analysis.* 88(6):1441–1456.

Perelberg, R. J. (2008) *Time, Space and Phantasy.* Oxfordshire: Routledge.

Rey, H. (1994) *Universals of Psychoanalysis in the Treatment of Borderline and Psychotic States: Factors of Space-Time and Language.* London: Free Association Books.

Rendell, J. (2017) *The Architecture of Psychoanalysis Spaces of Transition.* London. New York: I.B.Tauris & Co. Ltd.

Sabbadini, A. (1989) Boundaries of Timelessness. Some Thoughts about the Temporal Dimensions of the Psychoanalytic Space. *The International Journal of Psychoanalysis.* 70:305–313.

Schinaia, C. (2016) *Psychoanalysis and Architecture. The Inside and the Outside.* Tr. Giuseppe Lo Dico. London: Karnac Books Ltd.

Searles, H. F. (1987 [1960]) *The Nonhuman Environment In Normal Development and in Schizophrenia.* Madison Connecticut: International Universities Press., Inc.

Searles, H. F. (1962) The Differentiation between Concrete and Metaphorical thinking in the Recovering Schizophrenic Patient. Journal of the American Psychoanalytic Association. 10:22–49.

Steiner J. (1994) Foreword in *Universals of psychoanalysis in the treatment of psychotic and borderline states: Factors of Space-Time and Language* by Henri Rey (1994). London: Free Association Books.

Stilgoe, J. R. (2014 [1994]) Foreword to Gaston Bachelard, *The Poetics of Space.* tr. Maria Jolas. Boston: Beacon Press Books.

Tustin, F. (1990) *The Protective Shell in Children and Adults.* London: Karnac.

Winnicott, D. W. (1958) The Capacity to be Alone, *The International Journal of Psycho-Analysis.* 39:416–420.

Winnicott, D. W. (1965) *The Maturational Processes and the Facilitating Environment: Studies in the Theory of Emotional Development*, The International Psycho-Analytical Library, 64:1–276. London: The Hogarth Press and the Institute of Psycho-Analysis.

Winnicott, D. W. (1975) *Through Paediatrics to Psycho-Analysis*, The International Psycho-Analytical Library, 100:1–325. London: The Hogarth Press and the Institute of Psycho-Analysis.

Winnicott, D. W. (2002 [1953]) Transitional Objects and Transitional Phenomena. In: *Playing and Reality.* London: Routledge. (1971, reprinted 2002), p1–p25.

Winnicott, D. W. (2002 [1967]) The Location of Cultural Experience. In: *Playing and Reality.* London: Routledge. (1971, reprinted 2002), p 95–103.

Winnicott, D. W. (2002 [1967]) Mirror-role of Mother and Family in Child Development. [First published 1967] *Playing and Reality.* London: Routledge. (1971, reprinted 2002), p 111–118.

Winnicott, D. W. (2002 [1971]) Creativity and its Origins. In: *Playing and Reality.* London: Routledge. (1971, reprinted 2002), p 65–85.

Wollheim, R. (1969) The Mind and the Mind's Image of Itself. International Journal of Psycho-Analysis. 50:209–220.

Wright, D. (2018) Rooms as Replacements for People: The Consulting Room as a Room Object (pp.251–262). In: *On Replacement – Cultural, Social and Psychological Representations.* Editors: Owen, J. and Segal, N., Switzerland: Palgrave Macmillan

Wright, D. (2019). Spatialisation and the Fomenting of Political Violence. (pp. 167–187) In: *Fomenting Political Violence – Fantasy, Language, Media, Action.* Editors: Kruger, S., Figlio, K. and Richards, B., Switzerland: Palgrave Macmillan.

Young, R. M. (1994) *Mental Space.* London: Process Press Ltd.

Chapter 4

The Room-object Spatial Matrix in the Physical Space of the Consulting Room Clinical Study

In Chapter 3, the theoretical formulation of the Room-object Spatial Matrix was constructed, informed by Psychoanalytic spatial theory (Chapter 3), Freud's spatialisation in rooms (Chapter 2), and historical and anthropological materials (Chapter 1). Current psychoanalytic thinking on the consulting room was then examined, which does not usually distinguish spatialisation as a concrete phenomenon or identify that the 'transference' to the room could be separate to a transference to the therapist, but be related to a developmental theory of room spaces. This deficit makes the original study in this chapter important, where I will discuss the original study, to examine if the Room-object Spatial Matrix stages can be seen in the clinical material (clinical data), examples of which are shown here, with particular interest in the points at which the non-transferential stages occur in the material, to see how and where it could be seen to inform and aid clinical understanding in practice of the patient's clinical material.

Rationale for the Use of Case Studies

The case study is suited to my investigation of theory, as Robert Hinshelwood writes 'The case study is observation under laboratory conditions' and also that it 'brings psychoanalysis closer to natural science experiment than to psychological or medical research. (Hinshelwood, 2013, pp. 103–104). Here I am testing my hypothesis, utilising case material, which is like observing the consulting room under a 'microscope' (Hinshelwood, 2013, p. 97). Case studies provide the best possible conditions to give accurate evidence of primitive, pre-object material. In bringing clinical evidence to bear, Jan Abram and Robert Hinshelwood discuss, 'there are also laboratory methods for scientific investigation of babies, developed by Margaret Mahler, Daniel Stern, Colin Trevarthen, and many others […]. However, clinical listening to the conscious and unconscious expression of experience is the primary source for understanding the issues and puzzles arising in infancy.' (Abram & Hinshelwood, 2018, p. 42) They suggest that 'clinical listening' is the 'primary source' for understanding early mechanisms, so the clinical case is the

DOI: 10.4324/9781003188117-4

appropriate data source for testing for my Room-object Spatial Matrix stages formulation. As Jochem Willemsen, Elena Della Rosa and Sue Kegerreis (2017) write 'The clinical case study is clinical research *par excellence*'.

The Clinical Research Study Setting

The clinical research setting was a consulting room move. More precisely, it was two consulting rooms (and an interim room used as a temporary consulting room) and two moves of my patients between these consulting rooms. These moves occurred as follows. The original consulting room 1 (see Fig. 4.1) was located in my home, at the door end of my living room area. I used that space as my consulting room for 6 years. I explained to the patients 6 weeks before the move what would be happening, the time frame, where the new room would be (through a door off the corridor adjacent to the room they were in), as well as where the interim, temporary room would be for the 2 weeks building period. They were given a map of this with the address on it and the dates.

1   During a temporary interim of 2 weeks, my patients moved to consulting room 2 while the new consulting room was being built. This interim temporary consulting room 2 was located in a community building, next to a church, it was known as 'The Church Centre' (see Fig. 5.1, page 114) and it was situated a quarter of a mile along the main road from consulting rooms 1.
2   At the end of the interim, construction period, the patients moved into the new consulting room 3 (see Fig. 4.1) which, like consulting room 1, was in my home, this time in the room immediately inside the front door where the kitchen had been.

My rationale for using the period of the three-room moves as a setting for this research study was that in my experience of previous room moves, they create an increased focus on the consulting room. Spatialisation – the geography of the therapeutic process – is emphatically brought out by the moving in and out of spaces. There is therefore more expression of feelings and thoughts about the consulting room, and what I call spatialisation in relation to the consulting room to be observed. The two moves present an opportunity to observe the relationship of the patients to the three different rooms before, during, and after being in them. The setting for this research study, and therefore the material used (process notes), took place before the study began. I had no research question in mind when I worked with the patients. The work of psychotherapy and data derived from the material are unaffected by the study. The use of retrospective notes is in line with the recommendation of Hinshelwood (2013). The material used as data covers a period of 6 months – 3 months prior to and 3 months after the 2-week

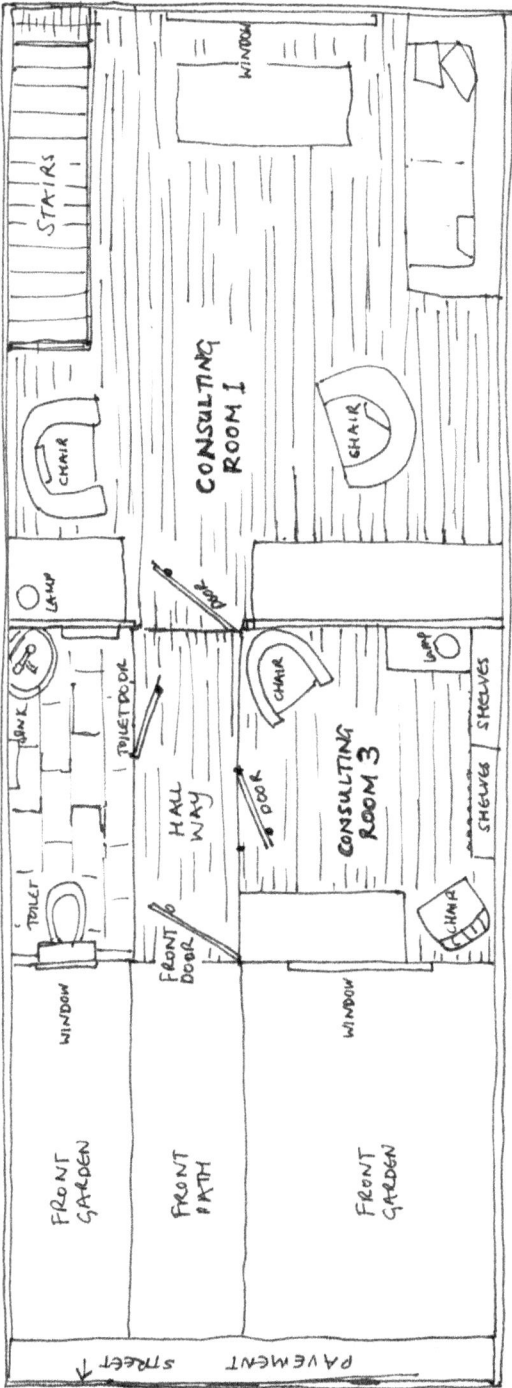

Figure 4.1 Original consulting room 1 & new consulting room 3. Drawing by D. Wright.

moving period. The period before the room moves shows material relating to the patient's expectation of the move and the new room, as well as their feelings about the temporary interim room for 2 weeks, and then from after the move shows their reflection on their prior expectations and their actual experience of the move and of the new consulting room. The criteria for notes being included in the study is that they make reference to the space of the consulting rooms or the room move.

Steps A, B, and C of the Study

Step A
The sources leading to the formulation of my hypothesis are- anthropological, phenomenon, previous residential and clinical experience, Freud's writings and object relation and Winnicottian theory. (Chapters 1–3)

Step B
Formulation of a hypothesis from these sources of the Room-object Spatial Matrix Stages (Chapter 3). My research hypothesis for the study was that: Spatialisation simultaneously involves a psychological projection of meaning and physically acting upon the environment, utilised to master the undifferentiated, relentless, internal pressure of instinct. I suggest that this can take place on a matrix of stages (that I am calling the Room-object Spatial Matrix). These stages representing a regressive, defensive function as well as a maturational one as a form of rudimentary containing mind.

Step C
Formulation of Operationalisation determinants definitions of when the Stages are recognisable in the material.

Operationalisation Determinants Definitions of When the Room-object Spatial Matrix Stages are Recognisable in the Material

Operationalisation determinants definitions are formed from each of the matrix stages in order that there is a clear criterion for how each of the matrix stages might be defined for recognition and identification in the material, during the testing of my hypothetical Room-object Spatial Matrix stages utilising clinical material. This includes approaching the material with a number of factors in the operationalisation determinants; the content of the words said the physical expressions and movements of the patient and their physical interactions with the room space as well as my own counter-transference feelings. Hinshelwood discusses 'using the recommended method of selecting occurrences by triangulation of content and counter transference' (Hinshelwood, 2013, p. 153). Hinshelwood discusses triangulation here as relating to giving at least two perspectives in relation to the data (material and counter-transference) that allow for a more reliable and secure interpretation, because it is supported by a credible exclusion of counter-transference distortion therefore there is more surety of its reliability. Paula Heinmann wrote on the importance of the use of counter-transference: 'The analyst's counter-transference is an instrument of research into the patient's unconscious [...]. From the point of view I am stressing, the analyst's counter-transference is not only part and parcel of the analytic relationship, but it is the patient's creation, it is a part of the patient's personality.' (Heimann, 1950, pp. 81–83).

Operationalisation Determinants Definitions Stage 1 – Primal Spatialisation

All spatialisation is like the original spatialisation of mother as an object from parts/part objects of mother/mother's body, and this action is re-enacted via spatialisation characterised by projection and action. It is pre-object and pre-transferential. **In Clinical Material:** Ritualised and one-off spatialising activities such as hand washing, chair stroking, it is non-symbolic pre-transferential and therefore characterized by projection and action. **In Counter-transference:** would include that the patient's feelings about the room seem separate, nothing to do with the therapist, the feeling that the patient's feelings about the room are irrational, inaccessible, and make no rational sense. These are pre-transferential, pre-object, primitive feelings. Also, feelings of exclusion, disconnection, no sense that the situation involves the therapist, feeling blank, bemusement or cut off.

Operationalisation Determinants Definitions Stage 2 – Room-object

Is an introjection of the maternal object and a re-projection in 'room', which can also be transferred to specific rooms.

In Clinical Material: the patient's talking about rooms that were either their original spatialising room (*Room-object*) or rooms subsequent to that, but before the consulting room that were re-spatialised. **In Counter-transference:** The patient's feelings about the room seem separate, nothing to do with the therapist, the feeling that the patient's feelings about the room are irrational, inaccessible, and make no rational sense. Also, feelings of exclusion, disconnection, no sense that the situation involves the therapist, feelings blank, bemusement, or cut off (pre-transferential).

Operationalisation Determinants Definitions Stage 3 – Consulting Room-object

Is where the consulting room is used as other rooms were used before as a direct displacement from one to another separate from the transference to the therapist as an object. **In Clinical Material:** It could involve ritualistic or one-off activity, including in the spatial array of spaces around the consulting room such as the toilet, hallway and street, relating to patients' emotions relating to the room which are unconscious or painful, overwhelming, and confusing. In the case of the move; obsessive fixation on the original room, high anxiety apparent inability to think about the new room, stuck, unreachable, panicking, and primitive feelings and thoughts that cannot be contained. **In Counter-transference:** The countertransference feelings are, as with stages 1 and 2 unrelated to the transference to the therapist (me) from transference: The patient's feelings about the room are separate, nothing to do the therapist, the feeling that the patient's feelings about the room are irrational, inaccessible and make no rational sense. Also, feelings of exclusion, disconnection, no sense that the situation involves the therapist, feelings blank, bemusement or cut off.

Operationalisation Determinants Definitions Stage 4 – Consulting Room-object + Transference

Stage 4 is the same as *Stage 3*, but includes the transference to the therapist, as the object, and therefore the room can also be related to the room and items in it relating the therapist as object. **In material:** Same as *Stage 3*, above, as well potentially relating the physical space of the room and the objects in it, to parts of the therapist as object for example, the cushion is part of the therapist as object's body and like their skin. **In Counter-transference:** Could simultaneously have non-transferential aspects of spatialising where the patient's feelings about the room are separate, nothing to do with the therapist, the feeling that the patient's feelings about the room are irrational, inaccessible, and make no rational sense. At the same time, clear countertransference feelings that what the patient is saying relates to the therapist and a dynamic between us, this might involve feelings towards the patient such as irritation, anger, guilt, or worry, and so on.

Operationalisation Determinants Definitions Stage 5 – Consulting Room-object + Transference, Outside the Consulting Room

Specifically refers to what goes on outside the consulting room after being in or whilst in the consulting room. **In Material:** Relating to a room outside the consulting room, that seems to be being utilised for spatialisation purposes, whether separately from or including the transference to the therapist. It may seem to represent the original spatialisation room, other rooms, or the consulting room. **In Counter-transference:** The countertransference feeling contain both the non-transferential, the patient's feelings about the room are separate, nothing to do with the therapist, that the patient's feelings about the room are irrational, inaccessible, and make no rational sense. As well as countertransference feeling give a sense that is transferential such as feelings of being excluded from the new room as projectively identified with feelings of exclusion from being in control of the room move process or the old room, envy, anger powerlessness.

Step D of the Study: Testing of the Hypothesis Utilising data set 4 – Clinical Data

Hinshelwood (2013, pp. 103&169) suggested methodology for testing theoretical concepts, using clinical material:

> The design consists of the setting, the logic (and research question), and the data. *The setting:* The psychoanalytic setting is highly controlled, and the technique precise if the rules of free association and abstinence are applied, if certain operational rules of prediction supplement clinical interpretation, and if the purchase on counter transference subjectivity is adequately managed. [...] in fact the clinical setting is not naturalistic observation. The case study is observation under laboratory conditions. *The logic*: Using the operational rules for interpretation [...]. *The data*: empirical data needed to provide the 'litmus paper' test of the logical prediction.
>
> (Hinshelwood, 2013, pp. 103–104)

I adapt this model, utilising the stages suggested by Hinshelwood; the setting (here the room moves), the logic (hypothesis and an operationalisation determinants definition of it for testing), and the clinical data. I shall track the appearance of the evidence of the 5 stages of the Room-object Spatial Matrix, in the data. In particular, I will demonstrate the pre/non-transferential aspects exemplified and where, when, and how these might occur. Jim Hopkins wrote that 'both Darwin and Freud claimed support for their hypotheses mainly on the grounds that they served to provide good explanations for the observations they had accumulated and could be relied on to cope with more' (Hopkins, 1992, p. 26) and that 'philosophical discussions of psychoanalysis have frequently focused on [...] how well psychoanalytic theories can be regarded as evidentially supported by the clinical data they are initially framed to explain' (Hopkins, 2013, p. 1). Hopkins suggests that Bayes's theorem be utilised where, 'explanatory hypotheses or theories are always also predictive, [...] the hypothesis (or hypothesized mechanisms) must perforce confer a probability of the data given the hypothesis is higher than the probability of the data given the negation of the hypothesis (supposing that there is no such mechanism) (Hopkins, 2013, p. 3). So, if the negation of the hypothesis is that the mechanism appears not to exist at all, then philosophically speaking in Bayesian terms, if my hypothesis can be demonstrated in the clinical data then it could be considered as having a probability of efficacy for further use.

I tested my formulation of the Room-object Spatial Matrix Stages utilising clinical material in order to demonstrate the matrix stages in particular the pre-transferential aspects, which open the way to demonstrating that spatialising into the room is not always related to the transference to me, the therapist, and thus evidence that the new view of transference is valid – and therefore an alternative to the standard view. The three patient case study examples shown here are from a sample of my private practice patients from that period, clinical material of which was utilised in the study. One male and one female patient, who I had worked with for a number of years and done several room moves with (Ms B and Mr D), and one male patient who I had worked with for under a year and for whom this was their first move (Mr C). This offered an opportunity to look at their differing relationships with the room, offering a wealth of observations as material. One key feature, brought out by these two sets of cases, was the difference in the patient's relationship to the room depending on the amount of time they spent in the room and how many moves they have previously done in them. In particular, whether it made a difference to their transferential relationship to me and their projection onto the room. I discuss this in Chapter 5.

Clinical Example 1: Ms B

At the time of the original study Ms B (there is material from Ms B, 6 years after the original study, in Chapter 6, concerning the Virtual Consulting room), early 40s, had begun work with me a number of years earlier, done several consulting room moves and had been in Consulting room 1 for 6 years. Her presenting problem related to early abuse by paternal grandfather, her relationship with her Mother as well as Mother's partner (from aged 5) who was abusive to Ms B. Her father left her mother when she was two. He had been addicted to drug and alcohol. She began working with me when she was 27. She had lived in many flats and rooms since leaving home and has no contact with her Mother. She had a good relationship with her maternal grandmother as a child; it was the only safe place she had to go. At the time of the room move she had moved in with her father, as a hope of a new start with him, and looked at beginning an ending of her psychotherapy. On hearing about the room move she had immediately made the whole event into a positive experience, mirroring her moving on with father and having a lovely home with him, as if, the act of moving into the new consulting room (and the 'adventure' of the interim temporary room) would make her move to her father's successful and defend against that being bad. However, during the period of the room move all of the meanings for the new room, as well as her room at her Father's, (their new start and her ending therapy) fell apart, and she had to find new accommodation, and stay in the therapy.

The Fourth Last Session Before the Move from Consulting Room 1, (lines 3–8)

She said, "I've been thinking about it; the church centre is a bit of an adventure so it's one sort of interim period. But that's where I am in my life. An interim space, what's important is my whole life is about changing spaces at the moment. It'll be my last room and that seems really important. I'm not really sure why. At the moment it's about things moving and changing environments, rooms, moving on. I think the room here is going to be a really, really, important part of the process of moving on, things moving on in a new phase, sort of doing it around me.

This is like **the operationalisation determinant definition of** *Stage 2 Room-object* **(from now on in this chapter referred to as '*Stage 2*')** where she is planning to utilise the rooms to magically compensate for the unconscious concerns about the bad father object (by re-spatialising the object- pre-transferentially stage 1) by keeping the good object father, at last rescuing her from the not good enough object mother. By creating the good enough rooms, there is a hope of at last having the happy family home that she had never had, now with father, and no longer needing the consulting room to spatialise into. **The operationalisation determinant definition of** *Stage 3 – Consulting Room-object* **(from now on in this chapter referred to as '*Stage 3*')** **is** a re-creation, re-spatialisation of the original **Stage 2** room as replacement for her mother. My formulation of the Room-object Spatialisation Matrix, was informed by previous material from working with patient Ms B. She talked about her relationship with her bedroom as a child, where she spent a lot of time and where she felt safe. She would rub her cheeks against the wallpaper which she experienced as comforting and said that she was conscious that this was because her mother ignored her the majority of the time (*Stage 2*). Another way of thinking about this, in relation to *Stage 3*, was that the consulting room had been a physically safe room space that she had not had in her home (apart from her bedroom of which the consulting room was a secondary spatialisation of her original Stage 2 spatialising). She has experienced this as a detoxifying space and hopes to carry it over into the home with Father (**Operationalisation determinant definition of** *Stage 5 – Consulting Room-object + Transference, outside the Consulting room* **(from now on in this chapter referred to as '*Stage 5*')**. In transferential terms (**the operationalisation determinant definition of** *Stage 4 – Consulting Room-object + Transference* **(from now on in this chapter referred to as '*Stage 4*')**, I was a detoxifying object which she hopes to re-project in Father. Counter-transference wise, I felt sad and left for the idealised Father, which she had felt with her mother in relation to her mother's boyfriend.

The Second Last Session Before the Move from Consulting Room 1, (lines 20–25)

In this session Ms B, after talking about it being the last session in the consulting room that she had been in for 6 years, and about the ending of the work after getting into the new room suddenly, as if she had not thought about it up till then, she talked about the patient chair, in which she was sitting. I had had the patient chair since before the first consulting room in this study, in a previous consulting room 6 years earlier, in which Ms B had been. The chair was a large shell-like shape in beige fabric. Although the new room was smaller, I was considering keeping it so as to least unsettle the patients.

> *Ms B said, "This is a great chair it's the kind of chair you could curl up and go to sleep if you wanted; you don't want to lose the chair; this is a special chair. We've had this chair since the old room [the consulting room I was in prior to consulting room 1 in this study]", she thinks, "8 years? So, the chair has already done a move, so it's important to keep the chair", she strokes the chair arm and turns and strokes the back of the chair.*

In her unexpectedly focussing on the chair and stroking it, she had unexpected feelings about the chair (her first reaction to the move that was not the positive defence discussed above). Faced with the loss of an important spatialising part object item, through the stroking of it, she suddenly became emotional: Tearful, seemed quite lost, confused, muddled, and a bit angry – This is **Operationalisation determinants definition of** *Stage 1 – Primal Spatialisation,* **(from now on in this chapter referred to as '*Stage 1*')** the creation of the object from parts of mother – which underlies all spatialisation activity as well as *Stages 2 and 3*, where her re-creation of the first room (where she stroked the wallpaper) in the consulting room utilising objects there (chair) to stand in for the original room spatialising. This could be seen in the spatialising activity of stroking the chair. My countertransference feelings would include that Ms B's feelings about the chair are separate, nothing to do with me, as if it is hers and need to be kept for her and her use of it (as spatialising object or part object of mother *Stage 1 – Room-object is pre transferential*).

> *She then said, "When I was young, I had nothing, no space, no things, nothing allowed in the lounge, here I am allowed in the lounge"*

Then here this feels like *Stage 4,* referring to having nothing in childhood where mother threw things away (including her bedroom furniture). There is a pressure in the countertransference to be unlike mother and keep the chair for her usage (spatialising) and also a counter-transference feeling of inadequacy (*Stage 4*) that she needs the chair as a top up to my functioning (*Stage 3*).

However, another way of thinking about this would be that her sudden realisation of the possibility of losing the chair, (representing parts of mother **Stage 1 Room-object**is **pre-transferential**) brought a disturbing concern about also losing the room and its function (*Stage 3*), and me (*Stage 4*) and so the stoking the chair was a spatialising attempt (*Stage 1*) and keeping the object going as well as asking me to keep it (as a defence against losing the object and for continued spatialising the object in the next room in it).

In the Following Session – The First Session in the Interim Temporary Consulting Room 2 After Easter Break (lines 1–6)

Ms B entered the temporary consulting room 2 and she said, "there are a lot of chairs", and looked around again "there are a lot of chairs to put things on, I'm not coming for the next 2 weeks it's too much – there's a tube strike scheduled for the next 2 weeks and on the following one after bank holiday Monday, it's too much to come back after a break. It's been really awful." She started crying then said "I just need to cry, the room stinks of damp," She looked around and said, "it looks like being in the 70's", then she cried really hard.

On entering the interim temporary room Ms B had experienced strong sensory memory associations. The smell and look of the room and objects in it reminded her of 1970s interiors, a period when she suffered a lot of abuse in different interiors. The physicality of the space triggered sensory memories of that and she felt disturbed and frightened. This is in stark contrast to **the fourth last session before the move from consulting Room 1, (lines 3–4),** above where she said, "I've been thinking about it; the church centre is a bit of an adventure so it's one sort of interim period. But that's where I am in my life". It is feelings of lack of safety and containment that she defended against with her expected act of entering the new room being an action related to her experience at fathers being good (*Stage 1* is **pre-transferential**).

The reference to, a lot of chairs, may relate to the fact that none of them are her chair (*Stage 1* is **pre-transferential**) that she thinks about utilising "to put things on" them *Stage 3*) but is reminded of the reality of feeling out of control of the practice chair (utilised for spatialising) (*Stage 2*) and the 1970s interiors where her mother's abusive boyfriend stopped any closeness with mother. This interim room brought up horrific fears of losing the object (Stage 1) and the consulting room (Stages 3 and 4). She defends against this by not coming again to the interim temporary room to remove herself from the dangerous feeling (in itself a spatialising act, Stage 1 as well as defending against the threat of losing the object – so here spatialising defends against losing the object so it is an origin spatialising enactment.)

In this example, it can be seen that the Matrix Stages in the material are moved in and out of quickly. The pre-transferential *Stage 1* material is evident in two instances where unexpected events; focussing on the chair and entering the interim temporary room, break through the conscious defences of the constructed positive spatialising phantasy about the move being part of the creation of a good home with father. This led to horrific feelings defended against, of the loss of the object, which in turn needs re-spatialising to keep it going.

Clinical Example 2: Mr C

Mr C, in his mid-40s, had been in psychotherapy for 6 months prior to the move from consulting room 1. His presenting problem was a history of depression and long-term use of anti-depressant medication. As a child he was close to his mother, who was intrusive and dominating. His two older brothers called him a "mummy's boy". He talked in the sessions about having no sense of ownership over either the space of his childhood bed-room or its contents – he can't remember having any things or toys except a womble pillow case. Mr C was unhappy about the consulting room move because he liked the existing consulting room. Mr C was building a room of his own in the form of a log cabin in the garden, and furnishing it which he reported to be his first-ever room, paralleling the work on the new con-sulting room. This relates to **Stage 5** and, as he began the work on it around the time of the announcement of the room move, it was a spatialisation project. This involved taking control of the room move process, by taking all the spatialising out of the consulting room either to temporarily hold it there, to defend against the breaking down of the spatialising of the object or perhaps keep it there if he felt the new room was really not good enough for the role of top-up container.

Mr C – Last Session in Consulting Room I (and Before the Easter Break) (lines 1–20)

He said, "It is my birthday on Monday and my wife and the boys are getting me a desk for my new room from Argos. Also, my son is getting me something himself as well. I asked for lightbulbs from the internet which are coloured green or blue". He was smiling a secret smile and looking to one side. My brother is giving me an angle poise lamp. It is worth £150.00" he smiles again.

I said, "Everyone is supporting you; that feels unusual".

He smiled and said, "There is a shop that does offcuts of carpet I'm going to get some. I'm going to paint a chair which I've had stored in the shed, I want to give it a distressed look, I'm copying that off the internet. I wanted to get a desk with locked drawers. My wife said we do not lock things in this house. She said that she has a rule that there are no secrets."

Here we see the chair which he upcycles and creates to be his own, is something like a creation of parts of mother spatialised (*Stage 1*) but here in *stage 5*, is a spatialising of a spatialising – a replacement of the function of the consulting room chair which stands in for the function of the original room, which is a spatialising of parts of mother. Interestingly, he plans to 'distress' the chair, representing his distressed object (mother) as well as an auxiliary container for his own distress.

He then talked about our coming Easter break, "We are back on the 24th, it's 17 days, it's a long time. It's the longest time, 9 days is the longest so far on the Christmas break."

Stage 4 – There is a lot there about secrecy in the transference, telling me choice things with a secret smile, so that I, like mother, can't take them away (unlike the consulting room) (*Stage 5*). There is also secrecy about lockable drawers in his replacement log cabin room. The counter-transference feelings are of being left out (perhaps a reflection on his feelings about the new consulting room 2 being nearer the front door and therefore further from the centre of my home as consulting room 1 had been – so he was pushed to the outside). The spatialising defends against his anger at mother/me and out potential destruction by it. Spatialisation in the room at home keeps the object going safe from destruction. Then he suddenly switches to thinking about the length of break being the longest time apart (transferential).

He talked at length about the room

I said, "Perhaps, although you might miss this space here, perhaps by planning the space of your room at home, you are extending the space in here a bit by extending it to your space and by describing to me exactly what you are going to do you are putting some of that into my mind so I can think about it and picture it."

I made a transferential interpretation relating to the room.

He said, "I agree with that. My bedroom at home was not my own; mum came into it all the time and touched my things, moved things, read my bank statements and things. I owned nothing. I only remember a Womble pillow case and I didn't own anything in or out of the room. I never had music or books. I just spent time there. Mum would get rid of things".

In return, his answer directly relates to the transference. I am the mother who got rid of the consulting room. He is also saying I've not allowed him to own the consulting room or anything in it or be attached to it. He had so little as a child and very little room to spatialise into **"I only remember a Womble pillow case and I didn't own anything in or out of the room. I never had music or books. I just spent time there. Mum would get rid of things",** he was very attached to the original consulting room 1.

Mr C – Second and Last Session in the Interim Temporary Consulting Room 5 (lines 1–25)

Background to the Session

The previous session had been the first in the interim temporary consulting room. He was anxious because there had been a break-in to the building where, at the front there was a boarded window and police tape. In addition, during his session, someone had attempted to enter the room (I later found out that it was the cleaner), the door handle had rattled and turned a few times as they had tried to get in. I had gotten up and held the door handle and the person had moved away. Mr C was very upset afterwards. In this next session, after me letting him in the front door, he looked very nervous and waited for me to lead the way.

He said, "I'm not sure where the room is."

He was looking around and seemed on edge and looked worried. He shut the door behind him firmly checking it was shut by pulling at the door handle.

This shows (*Stage 1* **is pre-transferential**) In the material: He looked very worried, he was holding and checking the door handle, physically pulling it (spatialising) to check it was secure and my countertransference feeling were of being totally separate form this experience, confirming that we were not connected, not in the transference relationship: he is in a world of his own. Also, since I got up and held the handle, then he holds the handle, one could say that he was not just imitating me, he was regressing from a failed transference mother to spatialisation. (*Stage 4* **to** *Stage 1* **which is non-transferential**)

He said, "I wrote some things down that I had thought about last session. The flip chart in the corner was in the group room I was in at the room at the library when I did the group therapy. I was also referred to it by the GP but it was in a different building from where I went from the one to one work. There was not a flip chart in the one to one room. The one to one room was in an older building; the one to one therapist did CBT. She didn't write on a flip chart: she wrote on a white board. There was a white board in that room"

Again, *Stage 4* transference (me also as unreliable mother for removing him from the room that he loved – the first consulting room). My counter-transference feelings were; guilt for bringing him to such a rubbish room and putting him through the experience and residual guilt about the person trying to get into the room the previous week, which along with the signs of the break in had really upset him.

I said, "It seems to be a merging of two memories it's reminding you of"

He said, "Yes, the 1:1 therapist drew a circle on the white board with words 'happiness' 'sadness' it felt like uncomfortable. I just felt uncomfortable. Not right. Something was not right. She was like a school teacher I was thinking. The [therapy] group room had the flip chart I remember in the therapy group that I talked about my friend's death and she [the group therapist/facilitator] wrote down words about it on the flip chart like a class and a school teacher"

Stage 4 – similar to above – this time it is an unreliable/untrustworthy/ therapist who he was within individual work and the room they were in. Again, it relates to my unreliability and possible harmful actions by bringing him to this unreliable interim temporary consulting room.

I asked, "how did you feel about that?"

He said, "I was worried about her writing my thoughts onto the chart and then it was to be kept till the following week and brought back out again and then I realised after that the room wasn't locked up and that anyone could walk in and look at the flip chart and the writing about the things I was saying about the death of my friend. It was horrible."

After a pause he said, "I don't like this room it reminds me of that feeling in the group therapy room".

This is **Stage 4 (transference)** it seems to contain previous bad rooms which are a re-projection of his original, unreliable bedroom and mother.

Again, a range of stages were moved in and out of, here, the **pre-transferential** *Stage 1* showing in the door handle holding and an example of *Stage 5* – the creation of a room outside the consulting room as a re-spatialisation of all the other stages, to defend against the loss of the consulting room, other spatialising rooms, object. Mr C paid great attention to the creation of his top-up to the function of the consulting room, room, and its contents, including his own chair (line 8) and secret drawers, parts of mother spatialised.

Clinical Example 3: Mr D

Mr D, in his mid-50s, had been in therapy for a number of years at the time of the room move. He had done two previous consulting room moves and had been in consulting room 1 for 6 years. His presenting problem related to early abuse and difficulties in relationships with women. His parents were from the Caribbean. His father died when he was a teenager, which was very disturbing at that time. He left university and ran away from home, thinking he had to replace father, and lived a lot of that time in hostel accommodation. After a few years he returned home and has lived there since. He is the eldest of his siblings and lives at home with some of those siblings and his mother. He feels that he is neither appreciated by his mother nor treated like an adult man. He owns a share of the property but he felt that he had little choice or say in his home. Mr D's home situation mirrored the room move when he was moved out of his childhood bedroom, by his mother, to make way for his baby niece. He then moved into an interim room (where people walked through) whilst building work was going on to extend his house; then, just as we were in the interim consulting room, he moved into his new bedroom, although he felt like it was not his choice, and he felt displaced and unsettled in his new accommodation. He struggled to settle there, but he was able to make something good of this and make it his own. He did a lot of work in the new bedroom to make it comfortable paralleling the work on the new consulting room. He cleaned it, creating a fresh space with boundaries and a lock. This was *Stage 5*, as he created his room as the new consulting room was being created. When he knew that a new window was going into the new consulting room, he cleaned the windows of his new room. This, as with the case of Mr D, defended against anything getting lost in the move process, taking charge of the spatialising for safety, therefore allowing a room outside to have all those functions projected into it. There is also a defence against the loss of the consulting room as well as his own (*stage 2*) childhood bedroom which was the original site of spatialising to top-up the neglecting mother, and who had just taken his original bedroom from him.

Mr D – First Session in the New Temporary Consulting Room 2 (lines 5–15)

> *Mr D said, "Because I've been doing something in my own new room, last week in the Easter break instead of being here I decided to clean my*

new room, or start the process anyway, I bought a small steam cleaner from T.V. I took down my wooden blind and cleaned all the mildew around the windows. My mum doesn't want them opened for security and it would make the room freezing. I cleaned each slat of the blind. The room feels so much better already, like the cleaner air I was reading up on mould spores. It's like I am taking over and owning the space. It's just the beginning. I'd never have done it in the past. Just like you are making a room. I'm making the room I want, to make it nice and new and fresh. And keeping others out of the room, making it my own, this is just the beginning. I cleaned my room till 12.30 am but I'm going to do the floor and ceiling.

He is not fixing a damaged mother, but he is inside a room space, mother as an object in space and with internal space, that was re-projected into his room to create this via spatialising (**stage 1**).

Mr D – Second Session in the New Consulting Room 3 (lines 1–30)

Background to the Session

Before the room move Mr D resorted to a defence that he had used with every previous consulting room move, where he considered the rooms were educational room stages from primary through to university. This had begun in the first room I had worked with him, which was in a building that reminded of him of his primary school and he used to use the toilets and go to the canteen as if at school. It was like starting education from scratch, with a fresh chance at it and the hope of a good educational outcome at the end. He had gone to university but dropped out after a year when his father died. This was a positive and progressive phantasy, where each room is an improvement to the last and therefore defends against any sense of loss. However, when he got into the new room, for the first time, he had an unexpected sensory experience of being in the new space, which brought very disturbing feelings to the fore.

Second Session in the New Consulting Room 3 (lines 1–30)

Mr D said, "Last week I felt very stressed getting into the room and it'll take me a while to calm down".

I said, "I thought about what you said about how you'd never see the old room next door again."

He seemed angry, he said "it's been very unsettling, it's very hard to get used to it".

This seems an unexpected reminder by me of something painful. I don't know why I said that; it was rather like poking a wound and there is something provocative about it relating to my own feelings of guilt about depriving the patients of the room and the upset it had caused and I wanted to get it over with (transference). Then Mr D's reaction seemed a very disturbed and distressed feeling of being separate from the old room (*Stage 1* **which is pre-transferential**). My counter-transference feelings were that he was cut off in his own world.

I then made an interpretation which could be thought of as transferentially leaning at the beginning, in mentioning 'my home';

I said "perhaps it felt like you were angry that you were in the heart of my home for 6 years, in that other room and since we've moved it's all very unsettled. As you said, everything was calm and settled for 6 years and then suddenly upheaval".

He agreed – "That's exactly what happened". He then said, "and now we are in a completely separate room. I still can't help feeling that I am in the head teacher's office and I've done something wrong."

He then thought about how we are in a completely 'separate room' which seemed to cause him more distress. As we are now in the 'separate room' but he is not separated from me, as I am in the new room with him, I would suggest that it relates to (*Stage 3*) (**separate from transference to me**) and that it is in fact related to desperate feelings of separation from the old room, and the pain of that as a relationship reflected the separation from his childhood bedroom/original spatialising room.

He then retreated into the phantasies that he had constructed prior to the room move about the new room being like the head teacher's office (that he has done such a good job of the psychotherapy process in the room for 6 years that he gets to go to the new room which is higher status, and then it will be like being praised for his work in the head teacher's office). However, here there is a negative spin on it, that he goes to the head teacher's office when he has done something wrong, this could be angry feelings towards me at having to leave the old room, like the head teacher, who will not praise him but tell him off (*Stage 4*).

I said, "You said that you never had an experience of doing something wrong",

He said, "No, only the time I fought back the guy who'd been bullying me and then I got sent to the Head Teacher, yes there was the experience of going to the Principal's office for being very good",

He moderated this with it only happened once, and then went back to his former phantasy of being good in the Principal's office (*Stage 4*). I then made a transferential interpretation:

> *I said, "Maybe you feel like you've been excluded from the family space, pushed outside, in to a special separate room and get less to see of me."*
>
> *He said, "Yes that was temporary, and I still had to think of the other room. But last week, when I finally got in to the new room it was like Ah! Collapse, then, Ah! actually got here, then Oh NO actually I feel totally muddled and feel I miss the old room and I can't think about the new room yet. Well, I'll be used to it in a few weeks, hopefully before the summer break".*

This interpretation (directly relating to the transference) seemed to bring him back to the desperate feelings being separated from the old room – **Stage 3 not transference** initially ignoring the transference but trying to rationalise that hopefully he'll be over this by the break.

Here he seemed irrationally disturbed and separate I felt very removed and bemused by his disturbance, as if he was in his own world. My countertransference feelings were that this was completely separate to me and unreachable (*Stage 1*, **pre-transferential**). Coming into the room was supposed to enact his educational stages spatialisation, but it failed and there was desperate feelings of loss and despair (and a feeling of desperation about how to proceed or indeed find a way to spatialise the object).

Then, in the discussion about the break, he moves to ***Stages 3 & 4*** regarding the idea of being without the old room.

> *Mr D then went on to say: "It would be very upsetting to see the old room next door now, I know it's changed, it's not the same. In my head the room next door still exists as it was that's all I need to know. I don't want to know what it's like".*

He is saying he has introjected the old room and, just as he had already spatialised it in his room at home, he cannot see it changed or it will be ruined. It may also be the way he felt about his childhood bedroom that now had his niece in it, but in his mind is still the first site of room transference **(stage 2),** first room-object and he also needs that intact in his mind.

> *I said, "So perhaps it does just feel like being pushed in to a room that's not your choice and massively inconvenienced in the process"*
>
> *He said, "Yes well, when we had the building work done at home, I had to have the room I was given, I wasn't given any choice at all (even though owning a share of that property)".*

This interpretation, although overtly relating to the transference, got a response of thinking directly about his first Room-object (**stage 2**) and how he had no choice to leave it, by his own mother. This is a kind of disturbing triple whammy. His unreliable mother makes him leave his room where he might spatialise to top up her functioning. His anger at her disturbs him as it threatens to harm the object, so he needs to spatialise more (his new bedroom) (*Stage 5*), to constitute the object, his Mother (*Stage 1*), his spatialising childhood room (**stage 2**), and the consulting room he had been in for 6 years (*Stages 3 and 4*). His anger at me presumable made his damage of me a concern, very disturbing for all of these factors.

Conclusions, Strengths, and Limitations of the Study

The strengths of utilising the room-moves for the study, is that there was increased focus on the room in the material and case studies covering that period giving an opportunity that is ideally suited to psychoanalytic research. The three cases shown here give an opportunity of diverse reactions and relationships to the room to be shown enabling me to test my model of the stages of the Room-object Spatial Matrix in terms of its precursors in early development of *Stage 2 – Room-object,* which I observed in analytic cases including;

1   All three of the patients in this study had experienced, during childhood, a depressed mother, who was partially, or occasionally available, sometimes intrusive, this being out of the control of them as a child and therefore evidence could be seen of the defensive spatialisation accompanying maternal failure.
2   Additional concerning, frightening, or actual abusive factors meant that certain rooms outside of the child's bedroom are unsafe (Ms B) or the child's bedroom is perceived to be potentially invaded (Mr C, Mr D).
3   Until being in the consulting room no room has felt safe (Mr B), this is then a precursor to the creation of a *Room-object* where the experience of some introjection enables some thinking such as parallel room making in a room space outside the consulting room.

Another strong point of this study is that the range of stage in the Matrix, whilst being in and moved out by the patients, shows its regressive defensive qualities and its maturational ones as well. Patients who are unable to utilise the therapist in the transference, much or very little, but have some spatialising abilities and some experience of spatialising into rooms can utilise the room. This, therefore, shows the importance of the role that the consulting room, in that it can fulfil, until patients are more enabled to utilise the therapist in the transference (therefore a maturational tool) a continuing top-up function. This makes the role of the consulting room particularly important, for some patients, particularly at the beginning of the work, enabling them to engage with the process.

In relation to the limitations of the study, although I have gained insight into the precursors of early *Stage 2 – Room-object*, I cannot see the patients, as children, and observe the actual relationship with rooms that they had in childhood. However, Abram and Hinshelwood suggest that: 'clinical listening to conscious and unconscious expression of experience is the primary source for understanding the issues and puzzles arising in infancy.' (Abram & Hinshelwood, 2018, p. 42). Charles Rycroft wrote:

> I should like to open by asserting dogmatically that we *inevitably* use metaphor when talking about mental activity. Thoughts and feelings, the raw material of psychology, or at least subjective psychologies, such as psychoanalysis, are experiences which people have, not phenomena which people observe, but when we try to describe them we are compelled to use analogies derived from phenomena which we do observe.'
>
> (Rycroft, 1969, p. 52)

I am compelled to use metaphor to describe these hypothetical formulations based on what I have observed and tested with the clinical material from the consulting room; however, this is the beginning of a process of study of spatialisation and Room-object Spatialisation. I have shown that my formulations can sit alongside the metaphors of Freud, Winnicott and Object-relations but have observed behaviour in my patients that cannot be explained entirely by existing 'metaphors' alone. I have tried to find a language and metaphors to describe what I have observed and to make sense of the patient's experiences. Utilising examples of clinical material (clinical data), I have provided evidence of the Room-object Spatial Matrix stages, in particular demonstrating the pre-transferential aspects. I can, therefore, conclude that I have established that there is a non-transferential component, which clears the way for presenting spatialisation as an ingredient of object relations. Possible reasons when and why it appears in the material are discussed in the next Chapter 5.

Figure Reference

Figure 4.1: Original Consulting room 1 & new Consulting room 3. Drawing by D. Wright.

References

Abram, J. and Hinshelwood, R. D. (2018) *The Clinical Paradigms of Melanie Klein and Donald Winnicott Comparisons and Dialogues*. Oxon: Routledge.

Heimann, P. (1950) On Counter-Transference 1. *The International Journal of Psycho-Analysis J*, 31: 81–84.

Hinshelwood, R. D. (2013) *Research on the Couch Single-Case Studies, Subjectivity and Psychoanalytic Knowledge*. East Sussex: Routledge.

Hopkins, J. (1992) Psychoanalysis, Interpretation, and Science. *Psychoanalysis, Mind and Art Perspectives on Richard Wollheim*. Eds. Jim Hopkins & Anthony Savile, 1992, Oxford: Blackwell Publishers.

Hopkins, J. (2013) *Psychoanalysis, Philosophical Issues* [Online]. (Accessed 26th May 2019). Available from www.academia.edu/4600503/Psychoanalysis_Philosophical_Issues

Rycroft, C. (1969) Model and Metaphor in Psychology. In (1991) Viewpoints, London: The Hogarth Press.

Willemsen J., Della Rosa E. and Kegerreis S. (2017) Clinical Case Studies in Psychoanalytic and Psychodynamic Treatment. *Frontiers in Psychology* 8:108. 10.3389/fpsyg.2017.00108.

Chapter 5

Discussion of Findings of the Original Study of the Room-object Spatial Matrix in the Physical Space of the Consulting Room and Implications for Practice

Spatialisation as a Defence – Controlling the Spatial Array in the Environment and its Implications for Practice

In this section, I will discuss spatialisation as a defence – how controlling the spatial array in the environment manifests itself in order to potentially defend against pre-object, pre-transferential feelings emerging. In the case of the consulting room moves, I, the therapist, had control over the organisational aspects of the room moves, as well as the building of the new room: The patients had no control over any of these processes. The patients believed consciously that they exerted control via the defensive phantasies about the rooms and what inhabiting these means including building rooms outside.

I suggest that patients defend against primitive pre-object, pre-transferential, feelings, by employing the spatialising mechanisms. At times, these were broken through with unexpected feelings triggered by unexpected sensory memories (particularly seen in the interim temporary room and new room, but with Ms B and the chair; Mr C the door handle and the room outside and its chair and Mr D with his own room outside, creating a primal spatialising pre-transferential experience where there is a panic about spatialising space and its objects being inaccessible or removed.

By way of concluding, I want to return in more detail to Mr D. I describe the spatial array between the rooms 1 and 3 and the interim, temporary room 2 including the spatial array of location, spaces, and objects within them and the layout around them. During the time in the interim room, Mr D demonstrated his worry about me and my ability to deal with the process (relating to his own anxiety and lack of control over the room move process), through asking a lot of questions about progress. There are several possible reasons for this, it was perhaps to do with a concern, that his job was to be responsible and somehow help me, the therapist who in the transference he perceived as struggling like his mother, and that he was needed as he had been by his mother to help. His worry may even have extended to mother's, and consequently his, survival. He worried intensely about paying his fee in cash,

DOI: 10.4324/9781003188117-5

during the time in the interim room, for fear that it would get stolen by 'youths' hanging around in the park as I went home, (a five-minute walk). He had also reported being worried about me getting back home, where the old consulting room 1 and the new consulting room 3 were located. His worry was spatialised as danger, in this insecure interim period, projected into, the spatial array of the street (see Fig. 5.1). The building work and changes were

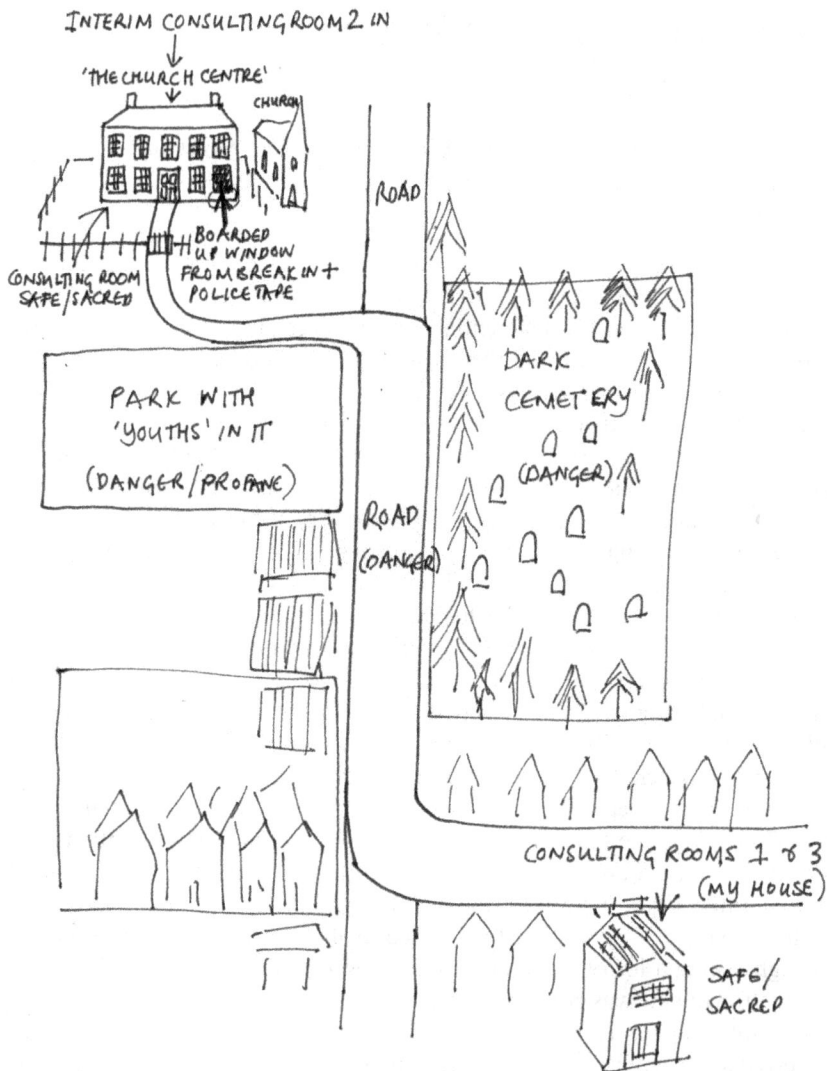

INTERIM CONSULTING ROOM 2 IN

'THE CHURCH CENTRE'

CHURCH

CONSULTING ROOM SAFE/SACRED

BOARDED UP WINDOW FROM BREAK IN + POLICE TAPE

ROAD

PARK WITH 'YOUTHS' IN IT

(DANGER/PROFANE)

DARK CEMETERY

(DANGER)

ROAD (DANGER)

CONSULTING ROOMS 1 & 3

(MY HOUSE)

SAFE/ SACRED

Figure 5.1 The spatial array of the street separating safety and danger. Drawing by D. Wright.

dangerous, moving from consulting room 1 was dangerous, the interim temporary room felt dangerous, even bearing the signs of danger in the break-in to the building, shown through the boarded window and police tape. But in this interim temporary room, even the prospect of the new consulting room also felt dangerous. He felt angry about the move and unconsciously experienced his own anger as dangerous. I think that the danger of his own anger, with no location, added to using spatialisation as a defence as a way of bringing some order and safety to it. So, the dangers and threats, whether arising internally or externally, were projected into the spatial array. This dividing up of the spatial array of the streets into safe and dangerous (see Fig. 5.1) is like the Westminster Abbey example (see p. 13) as well as the Nigerian village model, in Chapter 1. In Westminster Abbey the space was used, and thought about, to control psychological space. There were clear signs and rituals related to the margins of the spatial array; in other words, the parts in between – in this case that is the street, keeping the consulting rooms safe. As with Westminster Abbey, sacred and profane are kept apart to enable the safe functioning of the individual. In the case of Mr D, there was safety and danger in the spatial array of the rooms/corridors/buildings/street in between. Referring to the stages of spatialisation in this study, the danger comes from the primal, pre-object level; the defence comes from the projection of the spatialised mother. Mr D wanted to keep me safe, as I moved from consulting room 2 (the interim room) back to consulting room 1/3 (in my house). This involved passing the areas of danger on the road such as the park with 'youths' in it and the cemetery. This is also reminiscent of the Nigerian village model where the danger was all around the village and ne-gotiating the going in and out had to be done through spatialising – ritual and metamorphosis.

I have also suggested that psychotherapists can attempt to control the spatial array of their consulting rooms by copying items that Freud used in his consulting room, such as eastern rugs pinned to the wall and cushions, as if adhering to a magical spatial organisation designed for the spatial array of the room, by Freud himself. This might afford a smooth and successful passage through, and experiences in the consulting room, perhaps even creating the ability for the room to play an efficacious role in the therapeutic experience.

As we have seen, Freud created a spatial array with positive meaning relating to the potential for achieving success which involved the streets of Paris (Jones, 1967[1953], pp. 171–172) (see p. 44), Notre Dame and Charcot (Freud, 1961[1885], pp. 184–185) all of which were re-projected onto the walls of the consulting room in the form of the Charcot lithograph alongside his other 'Household gods' (Freud, 1961[1882], p. 8), see page 42. Perhaps this defended against weakness and failure (of actual Father), by magically evoking the education and genius of Charcot in the consulting room perhaps ensuring success for his and his patients' analysis. This could have been reinforced by the objects, such as antique figures, in the room. There was also projection shown in the dream (see page 41) onto the stair outside his consulting room. Here, as discussed in Chapter 2, we can think of this as representing paternal or maternal projections onto the spatial array of the spaces around and within Freud's consulting room. I will now go on to explore this further as I look further at the notion that Room-spatialising potentially relating to the spatial array of mother's body.

The Consulting Room and the Spatial Array of the Anatomy of Mother's Body and Implications for Practice

I have suggested in Chapter 3 that *Stage 2 Room-object* as well as Stages 3 *Consulting Room-object* can facilitate attempts to manufacture the holding and containing functions, through projections creating a rudimentary auxiliary mind and body space. In this section, I am arguing the case that the consulting room can be spatialised as the spatial array of the anatomy of mother's body and discuss the implications for practice of this idea.

As we have seen in the pre-object, pre-transferential *Stage 1- Primary Spatialisation*, parts of mother, part objects, are spatialised to create the object. Stages 2, 3, 4, and 5 contain elements of this, where parts of the spatial array in and around rooms and the consulting room can become parts of mother. In relation to the anatomical elements within and surrounding the consulting rooms in this study, that can make up the anatomical spatial array; there are the consulting rooms and their contents, such as chairs and blinds and (in the case of Freud, pictures and objects and rugs, etc.) toilets and hallways outside the consulting room, and the streets around the consulting room. These are all connected in a spatial connection of a spatial array of locations, objects, and their meanings and also their relationship to each other – good or bad. Freud brings imagery such as box, lock and key, womb, wardrobes, and cupboards representing the insides of mother, and the stairs, representing mother's body. He also showed items such as the picture of Charcot along with the pictures that are 'household gods' and the objects that can represent parts of the paternal body.

In relation to my formulation of the Room-object Spatial Matrix, when a baby is born, the things around the baby are the first spaces, the body, breast, the first physical spatial experience. There is the space of the womb itself, but how does the baby know that it is a space? It is all the baby knows until there is something to contrast it with. It is not a space, rather *a site for spatialisation*. In Object-relations terms, this is like part objects (such as breast, eyes, or face). The baby can cry desperately or furiously if the breast is taken away before the baby feels that its feed is at an end and that the baby then loses control of that process (and experiences separation). This would be because mother has decided that it is over, not because the baby has finished the feed, therefore all volition (control) is removed from the baby, which is distressing, disturbing, and disruptive to its continuity of being – the breast and the food are no longer available. But, in fact, the baby in its primitive thinking, does not understand the breast will come back next time. My understanding of this goes in underneath the premature finishing of the feeding, to a more primitive process going on – the spatialisation – that's the aspect I am bringing out and show in sharper relief. Spatialisation is part of the formation of objects but also defensive reaction to maternal failure. In the case of the consulting room move, it was like too early finishing of a feed from that breast at that time (that consulting room) when the patient was not ready for it to finish (because I, the therapist, needed to finish in that room). Therefore, the patients felt they were losing control over the room process (in this analogy: Feeding process). Mr C, Ms B, and Mr D, when the room was removed, had no control over that. The unexpected unconscious sensory memories that emerged were of desperate anxiety, perhaps losing part of the self, with a threat of disintegration or lack of integration of self. What I have argued it that the disturbance was the loss of the site of the spatialising of the object. This spatialising is a defence against the loss of the object. When the spatialising site is removed then it can be disturbing that the object cannot be spatialised and in addition gets damaged by anger at me in the transference for being the withholding object.

Returning to the part object, breast analogy – leaving aside the chaotic 'feeding' arrangement in the interim room, which was highly unsatisfactory and disturbing for some patients. Even though a new breast was presented for a new feed (and indeed for spatialising opportunity), in the form of the new consulting room, Mr C, Ms B, and Mr D, rejected the new 'feed' as not 'good' enough or not under their control. Mr C and Mr D put a defence in place, by making their own holding 'breast' elsewhere from introjected and re-projected elements, standing in for mother's anatomy, in the form of the *Stage 5 Consulting Room-object + Transference, outside the Consulting room.*

As discussed, in Chapter 3 (contributing to my formulation of The Room-object Spatial Matrix stages), see page 74, Ms B had talked about her relationship with her bedroom as a child, saying that rubbing her cheeks against the wallpaper and the walls comforted her. She had a sense, at the time, that it was to comfort herself because she felt distant and rejected by her mother. She felt alone and only felt comfortable in her room. Her mother's boyfriend was frightening and she was not welcome in the rest of the house. She used the walls of her room to stand in for mother's skin, hugging it as part of the anatomy of mother's body. During the consulting room move, her initially positive response (defence) to the room move, changed in the second last session before the move (see page 100), when, on stroking and looking at the patient chair, and saying, "This is a great chair it's the kind of chair you could curl up and go to sleep on if you wanted, you don't want to lose the chair. This is a special chair", she experienced unexpected sensory feelings of anger about leaving the room. She seemed to experience the chair as part of the anatomy of mother's body, (*Stage 1 – Primary Spatialisation*), telling me we must keep the chair, to retain consistency and continuity of the holding and feeding breast. In her anger she was talking about her mother taking things away and having no control over things. A lot of the patients, who are not part of this study, also asked me to keep the chair, I think for similar reasons.

Following this line of thinking, recall Freud's room descriptions, which I suggest relate to his mother's body, as well as his dream about the insides of his mother being represented by the wardrobe (see page 40). We also looked at this in relation to the Abbey shrine kneeling places (see pages 15 & 16) and the Chapel of Our Lady of Pew (see page 17 & 18) to get as close into mother's body as possible and as Figlio wrote 'I have argued that we are driven to know mother from the outside and the inside' (Figlio, 2000, p. 21). I suggest that pre-transference elements of *Primary Spatialisation* are a precursor from which the transference to mother's body was composed. But this can be moved in and out of at any time as a replacement for inadequate mother functioning by actual mother.

Another example of the usage of the spatial array, as the anatomy of mother's body, can be seen in Mr D's relationship to the toilet outside the consulting room. In the past, use of and nearby access to a toilet was always very important in different consulting rooms in which I worked with him. It is, however, important to note that the toilet was the consistent element in the move as it (and the hallway) remained the same (which was reassuring for the patients).

> *In the eleventh session in the new consulting room he said, "The toilet is so nice – a nice atmosphere, I like everything, [...] the towel is always clean, everything neat and tidy. The toilets at the gym are really disgusting, you wouldn't want to change in there. There is always a feminine soap smell here". He went on to talk about how his Mother's bathroom is always neat and clean and nice; and he's not really supposed to use it but sometimes he does.*

Perhaps the soap is a way of spatialising a touching and smelling of something 'feminine', mother-like, like mother's bathroom. Perhaps the sacred part of mother can be got near to, with things that can be touched and held (the soap and towel) that are like mother. He experiences his mother's body as benign (sacred) but her mind dangerous (profane) as he talked about his phantasy of whether his mother's mind can move through the walls of the house and into his bedroom and into his mind and know what he is thinking. In Westminster Abbey there are niches in the walls for monks to wash their hands, which, (as with Mr D) was a spatialising ritual, before entering the refectory from the cloisters – a marginal transitory space, neither sacred, or profane. Mr C prepares for the session before entering the consulting room by washing his hands in the corridor, which, like the cloisters, is marginal – neither sacred nor profane.

The Anatomy of Mother's Mind – Thinking About Thinking; Thinking and Spatialisation – Implications for Practice

Freud's observation of monuments in the streets of London being invested with emotional meanings to 'Londoners' (Freud, 1957[1910], p. 16) was a way of describing the spatialisation of feelings and ideas. I have argued that this dimension of 'controlling the world' is based on intertwining the physical and the psychological space, in which physical space can be used to harness and control psychological space. These manipulations and possessions of space are ambiguous: While they control forces in the psyche, they can also intensify the pressure for action against objects in other projected – locations. The less the occasions for and the more primitive the psychic level of thinking, the more there will be pressure to spatialize and the more immanent will be an acting out of the need to control the spatial array of the physical space and the objects in it. As discussed, this can also be witnessed in adult life, for example when under pressure. Figlio and Richards (2003) specify the scope and nature of the containing function of nonhuman environments: 'The role of the public utilities in the life of the mind must therefore be in an important way the creation *of* that mind, that is to say, their containing function must have been projectively invested in them.' (Figlio & Richards, 2003, p. 412). As I have formulated, in the Room-object Spatial Matrix, that the room can be utilised to afford a rudimentary thinking/containing mother function to provide a rudimentary containment of disturbing emotions.

When this is secondary spatialised (*Stages 3 & 4*) then the consulting room can also be utilised for this purpose as a replacement or top-up function (to be gone in and out of utilising, depending on need) to the therapist's functioning as the containing function. This is why the pre-transferential elements feel separate and cut off in the counter-transference, as, at that moment the patient is in their own relationship to the room and the room function. This was shown at the points of unexpected, unconscious feelings emerging, which were experienced as panic at the separation from this functioning. The sudden reminder of this function of the consulting room being removed, resulted in temporary inability to think and process the strong emotions/instincts which can normally be dealt with, in an auxiliary way, by the room, as a top-up to the containing function of the therapist. I suggest that this is a role taken up by the consulting room at times when this is required by the patient – as a replacement of, in the role of *Stages 3 Consulting room-object* or an addition to *Stages 4 Consulting Room-object + Transference,* the therapist's function, as an auxiliary container. The mechanism of spatialising, where thinking is replaced by action, is utilised to manage mounting instinctual pressure – the more developed the thinking, following Wollheim (1969), the more integrated processes of thinking and feeling will become. Wollheim wrote that:

> 'All such conceptions derive ultimately from an assimilation of the mind to the body, of mental activity to bodily functioning, of mental contents to the parts of the body. [...] It is not merely that we are at home in our body: we are at home in our mind somewhat as in a body. This, we may say, is the mind's image of itself.'
>
> (Wollheim, 1969, p. 219)

Wollheim is writing about the antithesis of Freud's idea of mnemic symbols, of the body, or indeed other's bodies – an assimilation of 'mind and body' and being at home in the mind. This is like the 'integration' versus 'localisation' that Freud argued for in his theory of Aphasia (Freud (1953[1891])) (see page 56). I argue that the more thinking takes place, the less there is spatialising (see Fig. 5.2). As Wollheim writes, 'we should have some specific view about the relation in which objects of mental states stand to the mind, assigning to this a positional character.

Diagram of Spatialising: The More Thinking the Less Spatialising

Here we have something like a disjunctive criterion for spatiality.' (Wollheim, 1969, p. 216). This involves creation of spaces, as locations in the mind for thinking. This is to accommodate ambivalent thoughts and feelings without having to split them, project them out and act them out in the space outside the self onto objects projected into and onto (see fig. 49). Bollas writes:

> As the analysand develops the capacity to think, [...] we may say that psychoanalysis assists in the growth of the patients' mind.'
>
> (Bollas, 2009, p. 39)

The psychotherapist may assist in the growth of the patient's mind, through their mind, being an auxiliary mind, and feeding back raw material; thoughts and feeling, digested by the therapist in their mind. This demonstrates thinking and assists in developing the patient's thinking capacity, as an auxiliary mind. However, what if the patient cannot yet use the therapist in the transference, has not had a good enough mother/primary care function to transfer, and has in fact functioned by creating the *Room-object* as discussed in chapters 1 and 3, where they have projected the holding containing functions of mother on to a room space? I suggest therefore that the role of the consulting room can be, as an initial one to the work, or top-up function to the function of the therapist, as an auxiliary mind space.

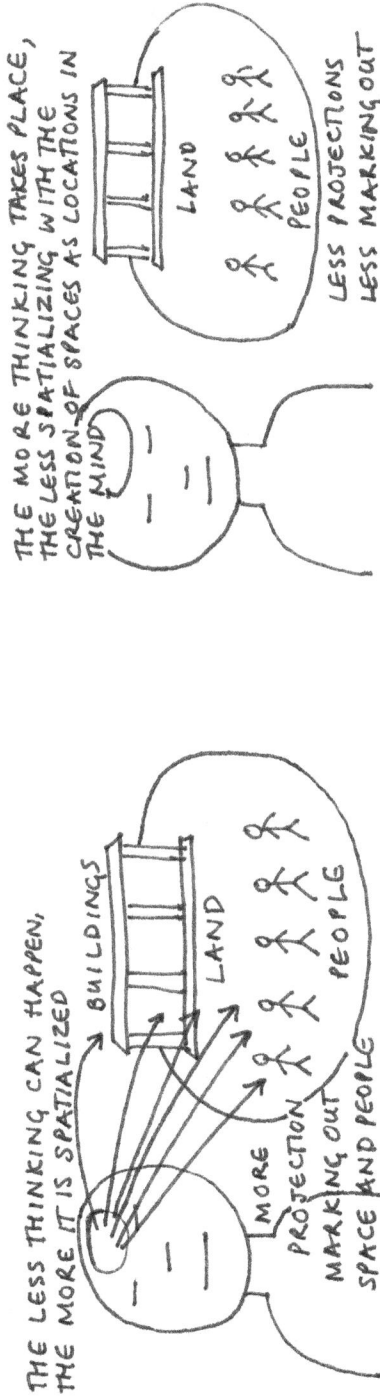

Figure 5.2 Spatialising into spaces, buildings, and people: The more thinking the less spatialising. Drawing by D. Wright.

Thinking about Transference and Implications for Practice

I am suggesting that the Room-object Spatial Matrix stages have, like transference, an important role in psychoanalytic work. As shown in chapter 2, Freud transferred maternal and paternal projections into rooms, but he did not theorise it. Freud believed transference was essential to the therapeutic process:

> the patient sees in his analyst the return – the reincarnation – of some important figures out of his childhood or past, and consequently transfers onto him feelings and reactions which undoubtedly applied to this model. It soon becomes evident that this fact of transference is a factor of undreamt-of importance.
>
> (Freud, 1940, p. 52)

I am putting forward an argument for the importance of the awareness of the role of the physical space of the consulting room when this can be ex-perienced as pre-transferential, spatialised, and therefore, have its own function separate to the therapist in the therapeutic process. It can also function as a separate or top-up container to the role of the therapist, as seen in *Stage 3, Consulting Room-object*. Therefore, thinking about working with this is also important. In relation to transference to Jane Milton, Caroline Polmear, and Julia Fabricius write that:

> '[T]transference to the analyst and the whole analytic situation, [...] give[s] valuable insight into each individual's unique way of seeing and relating. There are always little hooks to hang transference on, real features of the analyst's appearance, tastes and personality [...]. The patient's particular expectations in relationships, based on personality and previous life experiences, quickly begin to emerge. [...] The analytic setting is unique in deliberately existing to concentrate, observe and make sense of transference, rather than modify and dispel it. The analyst's position and function mean that he or she quickly tends to become clothed with maternal and paternal transference.
>
> (Milton, Polmear, & Fabricius 2011[2004], pp. 8–9)

I am suggesting that all of these ideas about transference can also be applied to the thinking about the *Stage 3 Consulting Room-object*. Thinking about this is a tool for use of understanding the patient's inner worlds, and if interpreted, the patient's potential understanding, as much as transference to the therapist. It was shown in the clinical examples where, at times, patients move in and out of different ways of relating to the room and to the therapist, some of which is transferential and some of which is non-transferential.

As with transference, the hook to hang the projection on is related to aspects of the room which may remind the patient in a positive or negative way of other rooms. The hooks are not just about the peculiarities of the consulting room that evoke reactions to other rooms, but that also evoke something of the original transference meaning of the room, that is, features of the original room that stand out because they stand in for features of the mother as well as of the room of the earliest experiences. Take the case of Ms B, who strokes the chair. You take chair to be skin, as an early transference from mother. Then maybe there is something about the chair itself. There must be a whole range of substitutions, from both mother and other rooms, other arrays of space and objects. As I have speculated Freud's regular changing of the prominent figure on his desk, his showing patients such as Hilda Doolittle (see Page 49) figures from his cabinet, his invention of the couch as an item to support the body of his patients as well as covering it with cushions and rugs for additional comfort, indicates different sorts of items for usage by the patient. This could range from the *Stage 1 – Primal Spatialisation* level of constituting parts of mother (couch cushions blanket for holding and containing the self) – a re-construction re-enactment of the most primitive pre-object levels of creating the object from part objects, to a much more advanced transferential use of objects in the form of figures (potentially maternal and paternal figures) on the desk and in the cabinets. We do not know Freud's intention with any of these objects in terms of hooks to hang spatialised room transferences on, but if therapists mindlessly copy the actual items that Freud was utilising, it no longer becomes conscious at all (if indeed it ever was) in relation to the meaning of the actual items for the patient, but instead becomes a spatial ritual from the therapist, meaningless.

What can be Learned from the Differing Cases Chosen Shown Here from this Study in Chapter 4 in Relation to Spatialising- Implications for Practice

Of the cases utilised in this study, Ms B and Mr D had been in several consulting rooms with me over years (and so had done moves before) and Mr C had only been there a year. Overall, I would say there was little discernible difference in reaction regarding the different stages on the Room-object Spatial Matrix – I would have hypothesised, that the two who had done room moves with me, would have dealt with the move more easily, as they were used to it and would have defences in place. To an extent this is true, in that, when they were told about the room moves, they were both readily prepared, defended, based on prior experience, with ready formulated metaphors (used before) for their relationship with the room, which afforded a defence against any unexpected feelings. These defences were concrete or hardened, having been, previously formulated by them.

Not only did the long-standing patients (Ms B and Mr D) build defences, just as did the recent patient, Mr C, but also these long-standing patients were sensitive to the breaking through of moments of unexpected memories, when unconscious feelings of disturbance behind the defence came through. They had both been in the room with me for 6 years, and one might have expected a greater attachment to the room and use of it for *Stage 3 Consulting Room-object*. Also, both struggled to tolerate the new room. Mr C, however, acted as if defence from an entrenched defence. He did not want to leave the room at all and, in fact, made all things relating to the old room 'good' and all things to do with the new room 'bad', a situation that did not change as he continued to despair at the loss of the old room throughout the material. It reinforces the idea that spatialisation is there from the outset, a constituent of object relations and therefore also a retreat to which one can return as a defence. As such, both new and old patients already have their developmental and defensive use of spatialisation in place.

Work After the Room Move Utilising the Room-object Spatial Matrix to Inform Thinking and Practice

Clinical Example: Mr E

Further clinical work has allowed me both to refine the theory of The Room-object Spatial Matrix and to consider its usefulness as a clinically-close, practice-close concept, in the spirit of Freud's distinction between metapsychology and psychology. This has included my work with Mr E, who I began working with 8 months after the room move in Chapter 4, so he had therefore not worked with me in any other consulting room, than Consulting room 3. I have found using my conceptualisation, of the Room-object Spatial Matrix of great benefit and help in thinking about and working with Mr E. who had difficulty with thinking and functioning both outside and inside the sessions. This often consisted of long stretches of silence where is can be experienced (countertransference) as if there is a threat of or closeness to some thinking and meaning that has been felt to have been gained and needs to be defended against, as too difficult, so gets destroyed. Often, particularly at the beginning of the work, there was a strong spatialising aspect in the room and at times it felt that the relationship that was contributing most significantly to the work was his relationship with the room itself.

When Mr E began work with me, he was in his mid-40s and still living with his mother and felt 'dead' inside, feeling he had no life, no career (although he had gone to Art College originally doing photography) and no friends. Mr E's described his mother as often following him around the house and talking at it him incessantly on subjects relating to her, such as her health, and he spent a lot of time in his bedroom (the original

Room-object space). His Father died when he was in his thirties, whilst he still lived at home, and he continued to live at home to look after his mother. During the course of the work, he moved out of his mother's house, a very difficult experience, leaving; his mother, his original Room-object space (bedroom) and the house itself. First, though, I will look at early spatialising in the consulting room from the very beginning of the work with him.

Mr E the First Session

> Mr E said, "I don't know where to start, everything is a mess, like a jigsaw, all the pieces are scattered. I don't not know what to say, this is hard, everything is broken up". He talked about living at home, "My mum is narcissistic, I saw it in a library book when I was doing research on something. She sees me as an extension of himself, I have felt like this all of my life, as though I don't really exist. I don't have friends or relationships, everything is a mess".

> He then said, "the chair is too low and at the wrong angle. I don't know if that is planned, I finds it uncomfortable and the cushions are uncomfortable, could I sit in a chair like yours?"

The chair he was sitting in was the original chair that was in consulting room 1 at the beginning of the study (see page 93) and then, as mentioned in the work with Ms B, (see page 100) I had kept it, although I knew that it did not fit well in the new consulting room 3 – as it was an enormous shell like chair of beige soft fabric, because Ms B and other patients, had expressed wanting to keep it (see page 100), 'Ms B had said, "This is a great chair it's the kind of chair you could curl up and go to sleep if you wanted; you don't want to lose the chair; this is a special chair [...] so it's important to keep the chair" and because I already felt guilty about the room– move anyway , as shown this countertransference feeling increased as the interim room 2 was such a difficult experience for everyone, and I therefore felt in my own counter transference feeling that I was unable to create a good enough space and I had to do my upmost to create a good enough space for the return to the consulting room 3 including keeping the chair so as not to unsettle anyone. We can look at this as a part of the *Stage 3 Consulting Room-object as well as Stage 4 Consulting Room-object + Transference* – involving myself in the transference regarding this. Mr E had experienced that the reality of that chair was not ideally suited to the room – it was too big and had to be sat on at an odd angle to the room. We could also say transferentially that he wanted the same chair as me which was more comfortable as an expression of his aspirations for the work he was embarking on with me reaching feeling more comfortable and an ability to feel more comfortable outside the room- and to change his 'rooms and furniture' of his own living space- to be able to move away from home and his mother. At the end of the session: *Mr E asked again "Could I sit in a chair like yours, where my face would be at the same height as your face. If you don't have one I could buy a chair". He then got up and left.*

We could say that this shows a Winnicottian potential for a true self act, which, although we had many sessions of silence after the room (and the therapeutic frame) was 'set up' enabling the silence to feel safe.

Although I was aware that responding to a request at the beginning of the work might be unusual – it seemed appropriate and in fact he was requesting a 'good' enough chair and **Stage 3 Consulting Room-object space** not only for himself but all of my clients were to benefit. In the following session 2, I put a folding wooden chair out for him in the room ready. I always sit on a wooden dining type of chair, as I find this most comfortable. He said that he wanted to sit in a chair like mine and the same height – so that was what I provided. However. as the room was small anyway and the large chair was still there, it had been somewhat jammed in.

> *On arrival Mr E said , as soon as he saw the chair, "it is really good."*
> *I said, "I am at a bit of a funny angle now,"* meaning if he sits on the jammed in chair, we are at an odd angle to each other. I was still concerned that I was providing a good enough space, compounded by the editions of the new chair.
>
> *He said, "it was a funny angle before and this is much better for me." He then got a book out of his bag, and began to talk about the book.*

Mr E seemed happy that I had made the effort to provide the chair he asked for that I had attempted to accommodate the space to be suitable but within limits of the space. He was determined that we overlook the odd angle as in a sense he had, or we had created it – in a Winnicottian sense, in the consulting room 'play' (Winnicott, 2002[1971]), or as the creating of the **Stage 3 Consulting Room-object** space. In the following session, Mr E also mentioned it saying that *"the chair is much better really"* and then, when talking about how people do not usually like him or notice him; **He said, 'I do not know what I do to make that happen.'** We talked about whether the new chair had made a contribution to the room, add to ideas, which were beyond his *"existing like a ghost"* and making an impact.

Meanwhile, I was thinking that continuing with the chair jammed next to the original chair was not a long-term solution, even if Mr E now liked it that way, as we had created it, as the overall face remained that the original large chair was not 'good enough' and filling the space of the Consulting room up. I decided to remove the big old original chair and replaced it with a cream leather tub chair. I had warned all of the patients that I would be changing the chair the following week to reduce the shock. Interestingly, all of the patients who had been particularly attached to it admitted that they thought that it had not gone well in the new room, and it was not the same as they had wanted, and that it would be alright to change it, even a good idea. When I told Mr E, he felt that things were alright as they were, and did not need to change now he was very happy with the folding chair (even though it was jammed in) as the 'transitional' chair in the 'intermediate area' of the Consulting Room-object space he contributed to creating would get changed and maybe ruined, as when a transitional object is washed, his requested created change that he was happy with, would be overridden. In Mr E's session 5, I introduced the brand-new tub chair. On arrival, Mr E said that he was not sure about it and even though he thought the angle was now excellent, and he thought it was also comfortable and at a better distance from me, not jammed in, as the other one was removed, he still said, it was not the same as the folding dining chair which he preferred.

Several months later, Mr E began to grapple with the idea of moving out of his home into a room in a shared house or of being a lodger of someone in their house. He felt that it was very important for him to be able to have this experience and to move out, although a complex mix of guilt and other feelings – fear, not wanting to leave his bedroom (first Room-object space) kept him there.. *He said, "I don't really know, I came with some ideas to talk about and it got stopped, stuck, shut down … my thoughts unconsciously got shut down. I thinks that I do that a lot. I was in a bad mood and I actually got upset about losing a room in a flat again so I may have been angry" … silence … "I came thinking about the special place I go and I wanted to talk about that."*

He is talking about a place that he goes that is wooded park and where he sits and thinks after the session – he depicts it as a better place for thinking than the Consulting room (Stage 5) so he can create a better space, but not to live in yet as he is saying he lost out on getting a room in a flat again so he cannot control or create that.

In the following few weeks he managed to secure a room in a flat as a lodger, in the session of the week in which he moved into it the new room:

> *He said, "It was far too hot last week. If you leave it until the last minute to put the heater off then it is no good, it is too smaller a room, it gets airless. I am not saying it should be cold but actually it is too hot."*
>
> *I said, "I am not able to provide a good enough environment sometimes". He said, "It is not that."*
>
> *I said, "But is like the chair not being good enough."*
>
> *He said, "Yes. We had this in the beginning" he became silent for a while.*
>
> *I said, "Perhaps it is not thinking about you in advance to put the heater off feels difficult like Mum"*

He said. "Well maybe … I think that I am not good at sticking up for myself and saying what I think.. I feel so guilty. My mum said to me, I hope you give me a mother's day card this year … I did … she said I do not usually, but actually last year I did. I got a card and present when I got her birthday present." He was silent. "I moved things out today, I was dreading it, I had to get suit cases down from the attic and walk past mum with them. It was terrible. It was awful, I took a load of things over today, mostly clothes. I might stay over."

This is **Stage 3 Consulting-room object** (upset by heater – not good enough, like the initial chair) and **Stage 4 (+ transference)**. Initially, he went back to his own room at home (original **Stage 2 Room-object space**) for several weeks through the week or at weekends, but eventually managed to move fully out. He lived in a series of rooms – some of which were a direct re-projection of not only his original Room-object space, but the whole house including a transferential projection onto the older lady homeowners that he chose to lodge with. Once he became more conscious of this pattern of Room-object spaces + whole house + transference projection to owner, he went for a studio flat – the best type of space for his developing self and he settled there for a couple of years. His mother felt that she could not cope in the house, without Mr E, and wanted to move to live in a flat, so her house, the family home, was sold, in order for her to live in a flat. Mr E experienced this as everything being lost. He took photographs of the house at the end, it seemed heartbreaking as if something of himself was getting destroyed, but also possibly freed up. His mother eventually had to live in a home and died – a series of losses for Mr E- almost overwhelming. With money from the estate, he began the process of buying a house that was extremely run down and needed complete renovation from top to bottom, although to get something affordable he had to move further away from his original home which although sold years earlier, he experienced as an extremely painful loss of the area itself.

In **the first session of the Virtual Consulting room move,** leading us on to the next chapter, Chapter 6, about the Virtual Consulting room, Mr E had his session by phone, expressing his concerns about the pandemic lockdown affecting his work and his being able to work on the renovation of the house that he was in the process of buying and whether tradespeople might be available. He talked about how it was not comfortable to have the session in the room he is lodging in as it is not private (the woman who owned it might hear) *"I am not sure about sound proofing in the walls here"* and there were technical difficulties re the camera and sound/microphone.

He said, "I don't like the virtual thing, its different from being in your house, its not the same".

I said, "You lost your room when the house sold, you never got your room back, you have never had your room,

He said, "No".

I said, "The consulting room at my house might have helped with that but you have lost that for now"

He said, "It'll be a while till everything is back to normal now ... I might not be able to carry on once I move – it is so far- this is the only space I have [referring to the consulting room] this the only place ... very upsetting".

He was talking about not being able to be in the consulting room (*Stage 3 Consulting Room-object*), or *Virtual Consulting Room-object*, (I stopped access to the *Stage 4 space* (+ *Transference*) things get intruded on by the woman he lodges with, and I took away the Stage 3 room) the loss of his family home, (and its location) his bedroom (*Stage 1 Room-object space*). Mr E is also concerned he cannot make a *Stage 5* space to hold over the consulting room, as Ms B, Mr C, and Mr D managed to do in Chapter 4. When Mr E completed on his purchase of the house to renovate, he was worried about the walls, *"everything is difficult, compli-cated. I don't really know what to do, I feel very unsure I don't know whether to take all the plaster off on all the walls."* And several months after that, when he was able to do his first video call, virtual session, the walls were again discussed *Mr E said, "old houses ... that is the whole difficulty- I am looking into what you have to do ... I can't do a course on lime mortar because of Covid".* This is reminiscent of the Figure 3.2 (see page 80) illustrating the *Stage 2 Room-object* space and the importance of the walls. He is building the *Stage 5* from the foundations doing it well enough this time.

Figure References

Figure 5.1: The spatial array of the street separating safety and danger. Drawing by D. Wright.

Figure 5.2: Spatialising into spaces, buildings, and people: The more thinking the more spatialising, Drawing by D. Wright. *Reproduced with permission of Palgrave Macmillan from Wright, D. (2019) 'Spatialisation and the Fomenting of Political Violence' in Fomenting Political Violence – Fantasy, Language, Media, Action.', Eds. Steffen Kruger, Karl Figlio, Barry Richards. Switzerland, Palgrave Macmillan. Reproduced with permission of Palgrave Macmillan.*

References

Bollas, C. (2009) *The Evocative Object World*. East Sussex: Routledge.

Doolittle, H. (2012 [1956]) *Tribute to Freud*. New York: New Directions Books.

Figlio, K. (2000) *Psychoanalysis, Science and Masculinity*. London and Philadelphia: Whurr Publishers.

Figlio, K., Richards, B. (2003) The Containing Matrix of the Social. *American Imago*, 60:407–428.

Freud, S. (1940) An Outline of Psycho-Analysis. *International Journal of Psycho-Analysis*. 21:27–84.

Freud, S. (1953 [1891] *On Aphasia A Critical Study*, Trans. And Intro E. Stengel, New York: International Universities Press.

Freud, S. (1957 [1910]) Five Lectures on Psycho-Analysis. Tr. & ed. James Strachey *et al. Standard Edition of the Complete Psychological Works of Sigmund Freud*, vol XI. London: Hogarth Press and the Institute of Psychoanalysis. 1–56.

Freud, S. (1961 [1882]) Letter from Sigmund Freud to Martha Bernays, June 19, 1882. *The Letters of Sigmund Freud 1873–1939*, 7–10. Ed: Ernst Freud. Tr: Tania and James Stern. London: Hogarth Press.

Freud, S. (1961 [1885]) Letter from Sigmund Freud to Martha Bernays, November 24, 1885. *The Letters of Sigmund Freud 1873–1939*, 184–187. Ed: Ernst Freud. Tr: Tania and James Stern. London: Hogarth Press.

Jones, E. (1967 [1953]) *The Life and Work of Sigmund Freud*. Harmondsworth: Penguin.

Milton, J., Polmear, C. & Fabricius, J. (2011 [2004]) *A Short Introduction to Psychoanalysis*. Los Angeles, London, New Delhi, Singapore, Washington D.C.: Sage.

Winnicott, D. W. (2002 [1953]) Transitional Objects and Transitional Phenomena. In: *Playing and Reality*. London: Routledge. (1971, reprinted 2002), p 1–25.

Wollheim, R. (1969) The Mind and the Mind's Image of Itself. *International Journal of Psycho-Analysis*. 50:209–220.

Chapter 6

The Room-object Spatial Matrix in the Virtual Consulting Room Space

I have looked at the use of Room object Spatial Matrix in my clinical practice in my original study (Chapters 4 and 5) as well as in the intervening years, and I have so far looked at two examples of applying the Room-object Spatial Matrix to the Virtual Space of the Consulting room – in Chapter 1 – Mr A and in Chapter 5, Mr E. I will now give more clinical examples of working in the virtual space of the consulting room, of Ms B (from Chapter 4 and 5), and new examples to this chapter, Ms F, Ms G, (both worked with me for a few years) Mr H (only in the physical consulting room space, twice before the virtual room move) and Mr J (began when the virtual room move had taken place) but first I will give some background on the Virtual Consulting room move, 6 years after the room move that the original study covered in Chapters 4 and 5.

Another Consulting Room Move; Move to the Virtual Consulting Room Space

In early 2020 events relating to the Covid-19 virus meant that social distancing was becoming a necessity and a potential lockdown looked increasingly likely. Therefore, it became apparent that it was going to be necessary to do another room move to a 'virtual' room as soon as possible. On 23rd March 2020, as things progressed with the Covid Pandemic, and social distancing became necessary, my Consulting room (number 3 from the study shown in Chapter 4), was not a big enough space to do any kind of social distancing and I spoke to my patients about the possibility of doing virtual work about 2 weeks in advance (not as long notice as a normal room move with maps and plans as in Chapter 4). I did a video call practice with each patient for 20–25 minutes in which we checked the logistics and they could talk about what it was like, with a view to beginning sessions by video call, the following week. The practice sessions were successful, for some patients rather exciting and novel being in a different Virtual room. As the consulting room was too small to set up a desk to have the session virtually on, I had to move back through to the Consulting room 1, that I began in at

DOI: 10.4324/9781003188117-6

the beginning of the original study, 6 years previously (see Fig 4.1 page 93), before the room moves shown in Chapter 4. I moved bookshelves from the Consulting room to put behind me so that the view the patients could see would include items from the consulting room to create as much consistency as possible. However, as with the room moves in Chapters 4 and 5, the virtual room and all of its spatialising connotations, created many kinds of reactions and I will be looking at these in detail below. I had learned from the previous room moves about my own propensity toward guilty feelings about the move, and how that can get in the way of thinking. My previous experience of patient's defensive usage of splitting mechanisms in relation to the room was also important.

Alessandra Lemma writes: 'Considering that the Internet and other forms of virtual communication have been in place for over 20 years now, surprisingly little has been written in psychoanalytical literature about their impact on psychic structure or the use of new technologies in the analytic setting with a few notable exceptions (e.g., Ermann, 2004; Carlino, 2010; Lingiardi, 2008; Dini, 2009; Bonaminio, 2010; Fiorentini, 2012; Kilborne, 2011; Lemma and Caparrotta, 2014).' (Lemma, 2015, p. 269). Asbed Aryan writes along similar lines; 'Working in psychoanalysis in the office or online, without preconceptions and without prejudice, allows one to de-dogmatize the setting, whether traditional or technologically assisted. If we become unduly custodial of the traditional setting and the regulating of the "correct" practice of analysis, we are employing a superego attitude to reassure ourselves of or value.' (Aryan, 2019, pp. 68–69) and that 'Psychoanalysis treatments, conducted online or on the telephoner, need our sustained attention to building a theory base if we are to continue refining best practice. (Aryan, 2019, p. 65) This Chapter continues this work of 'building theory', beginning with an idea that, for the first time since Freud's original first consulting room, the medium has changed en masse. As Gillian Issacs Russell asks, 'Will the consulting room be sanitary? […] I think that our entire future landscape will be inevitably altered including our experience and expectations of analytic therapy. However, I hoping that our experience of remote practice will motivate us to familiarise ourselves with the changes and loses inherent in technology use.' (Issacs Russell, 2020, p. 373). In this Chapter, I contrast the room move to a physical consulting room space in the study in Chapter 4, to the room move to the Virtual Consulting room space in order to show the similarities, differences and not only the areas that the Virtual experience is difficult, but areas that it can support and advantage the therapeutic experience spatially. Lemma has discussed the importance of being 'receptive to the possibility that technological developments can be used to support psychic 'development" (Lemma, 2015, p. 570) as well as the concept of the virtual, 'The virtual, as I use the term here, […] is an attribute of the real, an expression among many of reality. The virtual brings into relief notions such as possible, the potential, then probable, the fictional. Something is virtual when it exists in an not-as-yet-actualised form.' (Lemma, 2017, p. 16). Lemma also points out that 'As psychoanalytic practitioners we are nevertheless all too accustomed to the virtual nature of the real itself as it is filtered through a world of object relations – one in turn distorted by projective and interjective processes – that creates virtual others who carry emotional resonance within and inform how we experience and act. The analytic setting itself is a form of virtual reality too, we might say, as is the transference' (Lemma, 2015, p. 570). In my formulation, the Consulting room itself has its own spatialised transference – its own re-spatialised Room-object experience and as Lemma suggests this can comfortably happen in a Virtual Consulting room space. Yonit Shulman and Abraham Saroff write that psychotherapy can take place 'in any setting or situation' (Shulman and Saroff, 2020, p. 341) suggesting a vision of potential creativity in the Virtual consulting room. Carol Leader, also wrote that, 'The early weeks of lockdown in March 2020 were met with considerable creativity and adaptation from most of my patients and myself.' and that '[d]uring all of this upheaval, it was good to discover that, with modern technology, the work of the analytic consulting room could continue more effectively than I had imagined.' (Leader, 2021, p. 5). I will now move on to looking at how these challenges and creativities can be seen as similar and additional to the room moves viewed in Chapter 4, some of which will be shown to be similar to this Virtual Room move. I show here clinical example spanning the first year of the virtual room move, from 23rd March 2020, to exemplify how the Room-object Spatial Matrix can be seen in the work and helped me and informed my practice.

Clinical Example: Ms F

Ms F, mid-30s, began work with me three and a half years after the room move in the study in Chapter 4, to consulting room 3. Ms F's presenting problem was anxiety relating to her divorce and feeling of wanting to move forward and feel more confident as well as to feel safe and comfortable. Ms F is profoundly deaf, and as a child, did not have hearing aids till around 4. Her hearing made it difficult to feel relaxed and safe even in her own bedroom. We did a lot of work initially with her on feeling comfortable in her house on her making her house feel like a safe place. She met a new partner, and, like Ms G (below) moved in with them, just as the Covid-19 lockdown was beginning, and as we moved to the Virtual Consulting room. Miss F had the experience of missing being in the Consulting room, having to make room space in a new home with her partner, as well as get used to the space of the Virtual Consulting room. Ms F had the first session after the virtual room move from her car, parked outside her new home, so that she could make space to have the session. She felt that the car was an important remaining space that was hers. The following session was from Mr F's mother's house living room:

Ms F said, "It feels weird being here without mum here, I spoke to mum on the phone, I hate being here alone. It feels funny having this session in mum's house, I feel like everything is different about the work- it feels like last week working from the car was hard".

I said, "It felt exposing".

She said, "Yes it does, I am not happy sitting outside the house. Maybe I made a mistake letting out my place. Everything is different- I have to make space. The thing is, what room are we leaving all the things that I say in? Is it the car? That feels exposing, leaving things in cars, and where are all the things going to be left today then? Left here? That doesn't feel comfortable, it does not feel right (she looks and sounds worried) I cannot leave things here- I had to lock the door in case the neighbour comes in."

I said "Is it like we have the session and then it is as if the residual experience is left and might be seen by someone?"

She said, "It's private, its private I mean it couldn't be more private, I can't keep it in the usual room."

I said, "it is difficult not being able to get into the usual room, you will have to keep it here with me in my mind."

These are thoughts about how hard it is for her to make a *Stage 5* outside the Consulting room, the routine, gone and things feeling unsafe – it has been a very exposing sensory experience, where *Stage 1 – Primal spatialisation* has felt, like Ms B in the interim room (see page X) very distressing. The Virtual consulting room is very much the 'Bad' Consulting Room-object and the physical space of the consulting room – is the good one. There is also a bad *Stage 4 – Consulting Room-object + transference* element here as well. This is much like the experiences of Ms B, Mr C, and Mr D in the original room move with the splitting of the good and bad room – and in particular Mr C for whom the original room 1 remaining the good one. This was similarly the case in this room to the Virtual room, for many clients including Ms G and Mr H below. Issacs Russell writes; 'Little did I imagine that by March 2020, we would all be forced by Covid-19 abruptly to adopt technologically mediated treatment as the safest way to practice. We have had immediately to move treatment, [...] online. Our decision had nothing to do with personal preference [...]. Unsurprisingly, themes of loss, fear and grief have emerged '(Issacs Russell, 2020, p. 366). We could say that this was what Ms F was experiencing here in those first two session, that is; Shock, unpreparedness, and grief at the loss. Issacs Russel also discussed;

In my original research interviews [In 'Screen Relations', 2015], patients reported doing therapy from everywhere: bedrooms, living rooms, work offices, home offices, cars in work carparks [...]. An astonishing number of patients worked in bed under bedclothes. This is perhaps even more pronounced in the time of lockdown when patients have no alternative but to work from home. Finding privacy becomes much more challenging when people live in small living spaces with housemates or family always home. [...] I have written before: 'A bed is not a couch and a car is not a consulting room'. But now we have little choice.

(Issacs Russell, 2020, p. 369)

This echo's the themes in the virtual consulting room that Ms F was talking about in the session, not choice or space, in a car, but also not having access to the consulting room to put things into. Although, as with the previous room move in Chapter 4, I felt guilty feelings in the countertransference, for the patients being unable to access the room, my awareness of guilty feelings from the last move which helped me, along with the fact that, Issaccs Russell said it was 'forced' on all practitioners, to think about the question that Ms F asked about '*where are all the things going to be left*'. I did the painting in Fig. 6.1 and drawing Fig. 6.2, to help

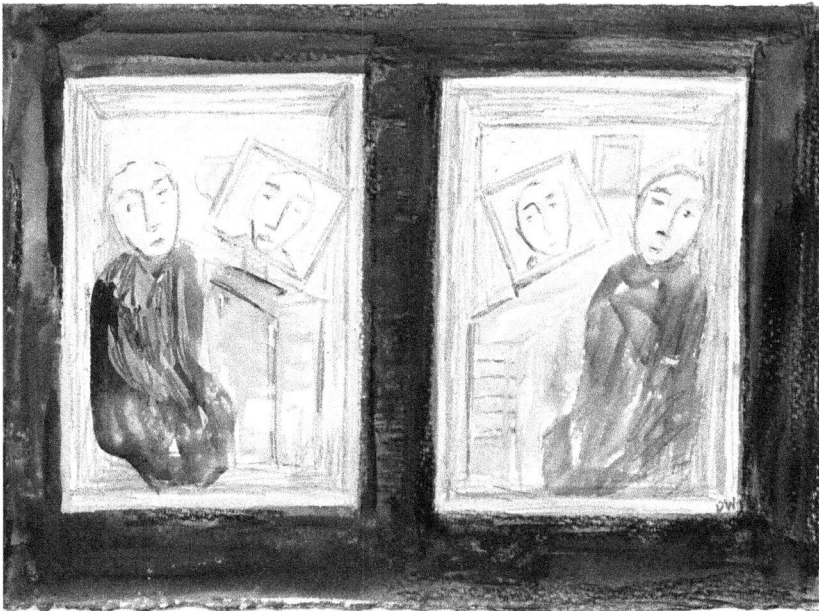

Figure 6.1 On-line working in room spaces. Painting by D. Wright.

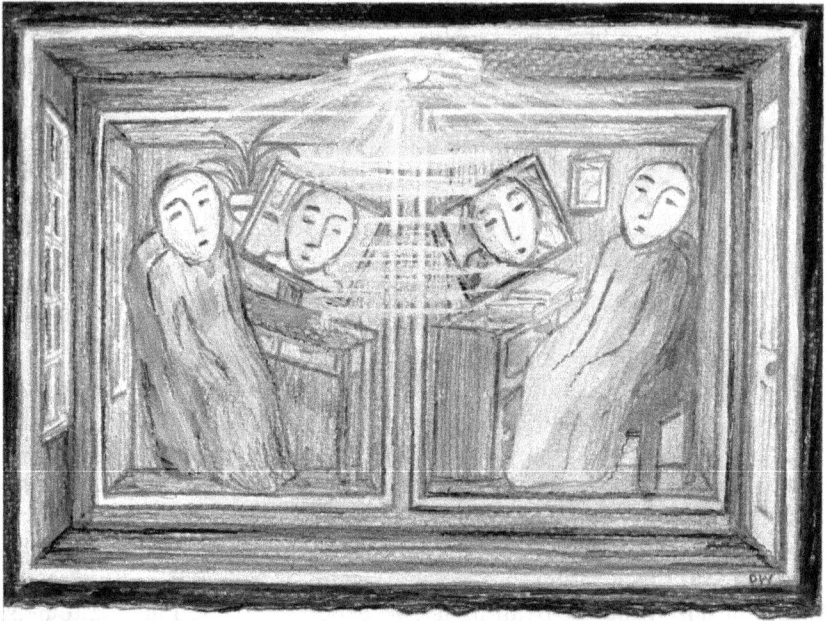

Figure 6.2 The Virtual Consulting room space I. Drawing by D. Wright.

me make sense of what Ms F was trying to understand about the Virtual consulting room space, so I could better understand it with her. The painting in Fig. 6.1, has a black space down the middle making us in separate spaces. The question of where *all the things* are going to be left when we are not in the room relates to the fear that things fall into a void and gets lost. The drawing in Fig. 6.2, shows a virtual room involving a degree of introjection of the *Stage 5* introjected Consulting Room-object space respatialised in the imagination, with a 'mirroring' (Winnicott, 2002[1967]) and an overarching containing 'virtual room' that surrounds the two room, which no longer have a void down the middle. Fig. 6.3 shows a *Stage 5 – The [Virtual] Consulting Room-object + Transference, outside the Consulting room* as an equivalent virtual version of Fig. 3.5 (see p. 80) in Chapter 3 (and the book cover) in the virtual expression of it. The internalised room in the mind of both the therapist and the patient is the room via the screen. In the following week Ms F showed me a tour of her new house and garden and talked about the new wallpaper that she had put up (which, as with Ms B, Chapter 3, 4, 5, and below, wallpaper can have an important quality relating to the Room-object, skin, and safety) that was part of her creating space in her new home with her partner, and showing me what she has achieved. At first, she felt unsure about showing me things

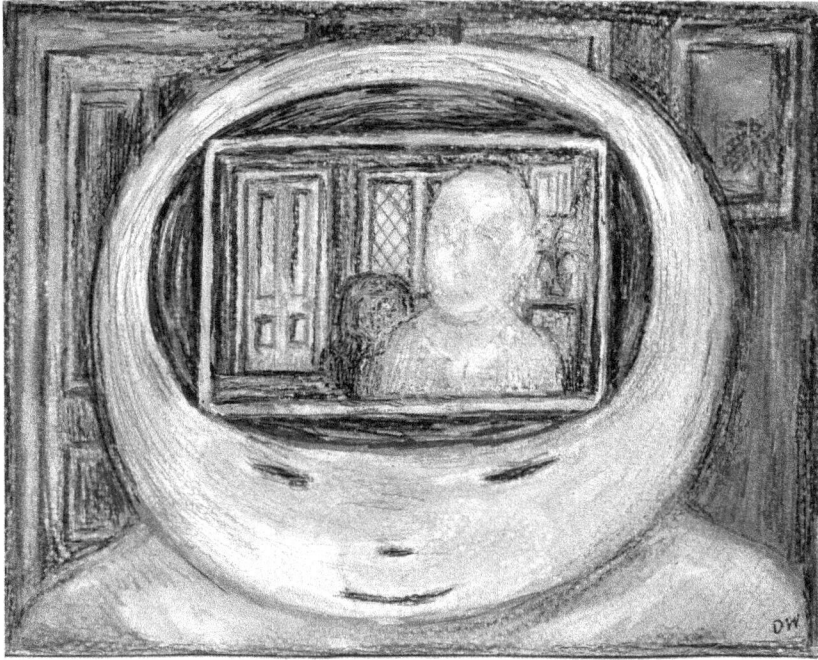

Figure 6.3 Room-object Spatial Matrix: Stage 5: The Virtual Consulting Room-object + Transference, outside the Consulting room. Drawing by D. Wright.

and whether my looking would feel critical or intrusive, which we thought about. However, she found it very interesting to show me things that she had achieved – a benign gaze that helped to place the new place for her. She commented from her own working on line, "*By looking at other people's houses you get more of a sense of people.*" A month later, she had her session in her mother's house from the conservatory, where she used to stay, she showed me round the front and back gardens and she showed me a picture of when she was young. There was an expansion of the spatial array of the virtual consulting room, in which a number of places were shown and felt safe, as well my having the opportunity to get a sense of them, that as she had said herself, gave an additional spatial sense of her.

> *Ms F said, "if I am honest, if we were going back in September I would need to think about whether I was coming at all- as it is still out there so if you have a lot of people coming and going, it is a risk. At first I thought I just wouldn't be about to have sessions for months and that was terrible and I never heard of zoom and I am not technical and now I am very happy with it and I feels really good about that and it's not perfect but it is good"*

So, unlike Mr C and Mr D in Chapter 4, she managed to change the 'bad' Virtual consulting room, to ambivalent to 'good' space and then a positive space about the virtual Consulting room, as well as her ability to create something of the *Stage 5* outside.

Eleven months after the virtual room change Ms F's session was from her mother's bedroom.

> *She said, "the dog is in the conservatory and if I am honest, I am not happy about it I was wanting to have the session in the conservatory. I am used to having it in certain locations now–Mum's Conservatory is one of them. I have to lock the door as it is hard for me to hear and feel comfortable and safe." She then talked about the possible changes coming after lock down ends. She said "Do you think everything will be normal by June? Is that what the government are saying? I do not want to go back the way things were- to 'normal' everything will change – I don't like change do I? It took me a while, about 3 months, to get used to the change of working then I got used to it. I prefers to work virtually now. I have got used to it, it feels safer I don't have to leave after and get home, I am here."*

There is something here about managing to create a home in the virtual consulting room that feels comfortable (see my drawing of this in Fig. 6.4) – a spatialised extended safe spatial array of spaces to be in, that I had been in the presence of and therefore the *Stage 5 Consulting Room-object + transference outside the consulting room* engaged in, in various locations, as a virtual safe. 'home' space.

Clinical Example: Ms G

Ms G, early 30s, has been working with me since 3 years after my original room move to Consulting Room 3, (see page 93) 3 years prior to the move to the Virtual Consulting Room. Ms G's presenting problem was binge eating, eating sweet products on a daily basis and anxiety – anxious thoughts with some OCD thoughts and behaviours. Ms G's mother had been critically ill with cancer for a number of years, which Ms G felt had started the binge eating and anxiety. Ms G was very close to her mother and she felt that she needed support in the work to deal with supporting her mother, the stress of the illness (and her anxiety and binge eating) as well as wanting support to be more separate and independent from her mother, while she had the chance, and to prepare for losing her mother. In her early childhood, she remembered that when her mother's best friend came round, they used to chat a lot and Ms G "hated it" and felt left out. Also, if her parents had their friends round or went out she felt "really excluded". Whilst in her mid-teenage years, Ms G had supported her mother, through a time when her

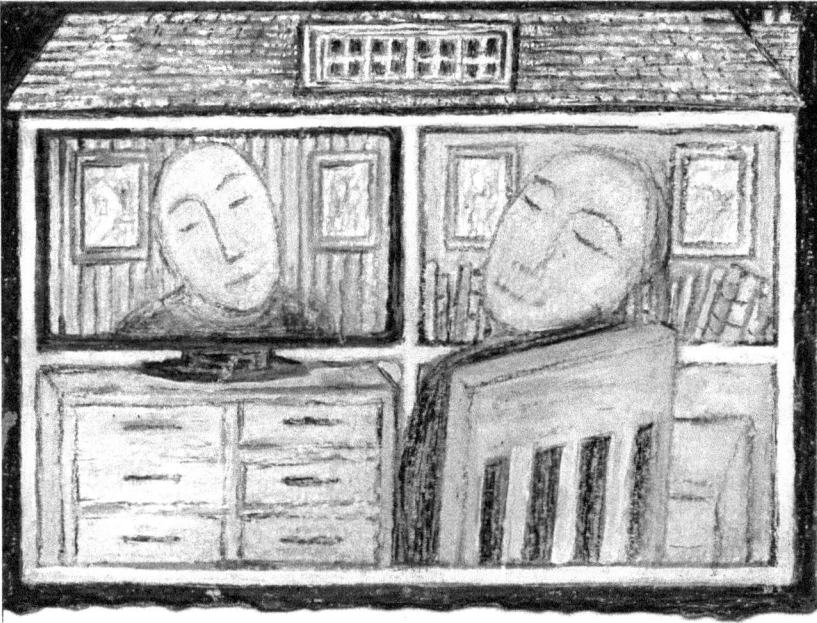

Figure 6.4 Home from Home; The Virtual Consulting room space III. Drawing by
    D. Wright.

Dad had had an affair (which felt like a heavy burden to her at the age
of 13). However, once her mother and father were reconciled – they moved
away to start a new life, leaving Ms G feeling left behind, even though she
had lived independently of her parents for 2 year. She felt that at times her
father colonised her mother and it was hard to access her. A particular in-
stance of this is when her mother and father were on holiday and her mother
would not take a mobile phone and her father would not pass his phone
over. It felt that access to her mother was controlled by him. This became a
screen memory in our work which was used to think about times when her
mother, is inaccessible, or me, then during the virtual consulting room move,
the physical space of Consulting room was inaccessible. Ms G's Mother had
passed away a year into the work, and she had made the best use of the time
to think about her relationship with her mother and begin the separation
and independence process, although it was felt to be an ongoing process,
encompassing growing up and potentially wanting her own family.

In a session a few weeks after Ms G's Mother has passed away:

*Ms G said sadly, "I loved her really she was a wonderful person, it's so
unfair that she has gone, she should not have been taken it is so unfair".*

I said, "that is a familiar feeling when she was taken away by your dad to live on the coast".

Ms G said, "she wasn't taken she went"

I said, "That feels like an angry feeling".

Ms G is thinking here of being taken by Dad, taken from her, not having access to her and her mother wanting to go – this is layers of anger of loss of Mum, spaces, and places.

Ms G agreed then went on to talk about visiting her parent's house, "it is not exciting like when I went to Mum's house. It is not exciting. It's not the same as my relationship with dad. I used to tell mum everything. I arrived feeling fed up. Mum is not there. He wants to get rid of her hand bags as well, it was really upsetting. And clear the wardrobe."

It is interesting that she refers to the house as "Mum's" and that things of hers are being removed.

The Virtual Consulting Room Move

Two years after this, Ms G had managed to separate and move forward and began a relationship. Like Ms F, at the point of the Virtual consulting room move, she had just moved in with her new partner, a situation, that, though it would have happened anyway, like Ms F, was partially speeded up by the impending Covid-related lockdown process.

Ms G – First Session After the Move to the Virtual Room (from the Bedroom in her Partner's Flat where She has Moved in to)

Ms G talked about the video call practice that we did at the end of the previous week- and how it was fine as she does a lot of video calls at work and that although her new partner was there, in the back ground, she explained, "that doesn't matter and it was just a practice- it is his flat, and we spend a lot of time in the living room, we both work in there and this is the bedroom," she gestured around the room, "I was through there for the practice – but obviously I will come in here for the session and he not to come in or listen." She was talking in a low tone though.

Ms G then showed me the bedroom, the walls, the shelves, the window and the large canvas photograph of her mother that she had put on the wall that featured in the back ground of the session to one side. She went on to talk about moving into this flat the previous week, and living there, she said that she is very happy to be there but that she feels upset that her mother cannot see this flat.

Suddenly the door opened and her partner walked in and went to the drawers to get something out.

Here Ms G's attempt at creating a *Stage 5* space that is suitable for the sessions felt horribly intruded on, in a very sensory shocking way, that we can think of as a *Stage 1 – Primal spatialisation* experience, which we could say was Stage 1, whilst also being a separation from *Stage 2* Safe Room-object, a separation from *Stage 4 Consulting-room object + Transference*, and the attempt to create a *Stage 5* space.

Ms G – Second Session After the Virtual Room Move (From Ms G's Car)

Ms G talked about what happened in the last session, and how distressing it was- how angry she felt- "having the session in the car- feels safer, I was really angry last week, I still feel angry … when will things get back to normal? Have you had any indication of when I can come back?"

We thought a great deal over the next weeks about the feeling of intrusion on the space with us, (*Stage 4 + Transference*), and her inability to access the consulting room, like the screen memory of Dad taking Mum away on holiday and her not getting access on the phone. She continued to ask the following week *"When will I come back?"* (which countertransferentially felt like depriving her of access to the room reminiscent of the room moves in Chapter 4).

Ms G found engaging in the Virtual consulting room, helped by the medium of emailing, which became a spatialising part of the virtual room, for her and other patients. Creating a routine, I emailed everyone at the same time at the beginning of every week, with all the zoom links for the week. Ms G always gave small email replies to these, which, along with occasional emails about a session arrangement, quickly became part of the Virtual consulting room communication frame. I suggest that because the text of an email takes place across the same screen that the video calls take place on, it could be thought of as 'topping up' up the session/virtual room experience by creating an additional interaction that, although is in typed words, is on the same screen/room space, so becomes part of the virtual room space. For Ms G this becomes an important bridge to me in my room that is private and does not feel intruded on. This could be like the attempt to text her mother whilst she is on holiday. Horst Kachele writes that, 'Email communications can facilitate the establishment of an alliance that supports a therapeutic relationship' (Kachele, 2019, p. 49) and Vincent et al. write about Therapist's use of emails where; 'emails with a client between sessions as a way of containing his otherwise unmanageable feelings.' (Vincent et al, 2017, p. 68) We could say here that email supported the Virtual Room move by provide an additional accessible element to the Virtual consulting Room, and therefore was a feature of the Virtual consulting room. Interestingly, Liliana Manguel writes: 'When we speak of teleanalysis, also referred to as distance psychoanalysis and remote psychoanalysis, we begin to con-template the experience of nearness and distance and feeling close or far away.[…] in my opinion, the sense of closeness in the analytic pair does not necessarily depend on physical proximity. What is essential for the sense of closeness in a true encounter. Reading Freud's letters to Fliess, it is clear that, without meeting as embodied minds in the same room, Freud and Fliess maintained such a true encounter. Freud invested his trust in Fliess, and Fliess was privileged to receive and respond to his epistolary commu-nications about dream life and family and professional circumstances. Nowadays typed emails and online verbal communications take the place of handwritten letters as devices for bringing the distance between people in different locations. A similarly close encounter is possible using technology. (Manguel, 2019, p. 90) This is a fascinating reference to Freud's own practice and his virtual analysis experience via letter that transcended clo-seness and distance. Email, as we have seen with the 'screen share' feature discussed by with Jordan Bate and Norka Malberg (2020) and Yonit Shulman & Abraham Saroff (2020), in Chapter 1 in the case of Mr A, is an additional feature of the Virtual consulting room space.

After 3 months of the lockdown, living with her new partner, they decide to move to her house that was bigger and with a spare room. In the session before moving, she said at the end of session – *"doing the sessions via zoom is 90% as effective as the room"* – which was also perhaps that the flat had been 90% effective as a home. As with Ms F, this was a move away from the split up bad virtual consulting Room-object to something more balanced. Interestingly, in the following session, after they had just moved into her house, Ms G said that she felt that *"the work is 99% effective as it was before lock down face to face."* So, it had increased effectiveness by 9% in the move to her house; perhaps, again it is a spatialised way of saying that being in her house and space is 9% more effective and having the spare room to have the sessions is then became very important, but it is also clear that in spatialising terms the spare room in her house is important for other reasons.

In the following session, she showed me how she had converted her spare room to an office and space to have her session:

Ms G said, "Mum stayed in the spare room, she used to sleep on this bed, [she shows me by moving the computer screen around]. We are taking away the mattress she slept on, changing the room and the house, she was on the sofa though as well. I have ordered a new chair for my desk"

Ms G then showed me the things on her new desk- a buddha and desk accessories, desk, and then said, "I am a lot happier having the session in the spare room than in his flat. I really did not like the car. I still says for him to wear headphones- but it feels like there is more space in this house as it is physically bigger and I can shut the door, this feels like a safe space in here.

Making the *Stage 5* space to have the sessions in, was helped greatly by it being in the room that mum stayed in, as the sensory memories in spatialising terms were related to the space of her mother, mother's body, and the space around it, which meant that all of the element to create a Virtual consulting room through the *Stage 5 – Consulting Room-object + transference outside the consulting room* were enhanced.

Further Clinical Example: Ms B

Ms B, as discuss on p. 98, had been mainly doing session by phone in the previous 2 years due to a moving to her new flat a distance away. The room move to the virtual consulting room had revolutionary opportunities in various ways, but before looking at that we will first look briefly at a session 2 years after the original room in Chapter 4, after Ms B moved into her new flat and was having some decorating done including putting up the living room wallpaper (featured later in my drawing, Fig. 6.5).

Ms B was very upset and distressed, she said, "I was so upset. The guy came in and there was lots of trouble about the start time. He took four hours, then he rang and I said I will put the money through, but I will come back. When I arrived back there was bits missing off the wall paper, paint had gone onto the ceiling and on décor not needing done. I was really upset. I said to my brother I would rather have paid £1000 to know it would be better and he said that is no guarantee it would be any better."

I said, "It feels so intrusive, on your walls and your space"

Ms B said, "Yes it does, I can put things right with the wallpaper and ceiling myself. But is feels like he has had a shower, he has been everywhere, I gave him the money to get rid of him, I don't want him back in my flat."

Her new flat had felt violated and intruded on which would be a direct relation to the original **Stage 2 Room-object** space (bad room space) see Chapter 4 Page 101, and discussed in Chapter 5. She wanted to create a different kind of Room-object space, (one that did not feel intruded on like her original *Stage 2 Room-object* spaces (which still appear in her dreams) including new wallpaper (which in Fig. 3.2, p. 80, had the association with skin). In later re-spatialised Room-objects rooms, there were grubs in the mattress in one room in a flat, or in another a cockroach infestation. Ms B was attempting to make a *Stage 5* room space that also contained the consulting room space and me in the transference, to keep it safe and contained.

In the following session:

> *Ms B said, "I am fed up, I try to make good things and they go wrong. More things have gone wrong. Since the guy left, I have found that there is a light bulb missing out of my bedroom, dents in the wall and bits dented in front of the door. I am very, very upset and angry. It feels like the house has been abused. I feel humiliated. I really made the wrong choice about him. No one cares. I talked to my brother and he is going on holiday with mum, he doesn't care, no one cares about me. You are not a real person and I can't meet up with you, you are not a real relationship, but you are the only person who knows what is going on."*

> *I said, "That feels painful."*

> *Ms B, "It's awful, I am fed up coming, it is such a long journey now I have moved here. I want to do phone sessions here from my flat. In want to stay here."*

Ms B was trying to create her own *Stage 5* space (her first safe space) and somehow merge it with the consulting room by having the session there for fear of something getting violated again if she leaves, and to shore up the flat's defences to protect the space and holding space to protect her. The phone session arrangement, with some in-room session continued until the Virtual room move occurred. At first the prospect of doing a video call session felt potentially intrusive, like Ms F, and she stayed with having her session on the phone bringing the following dream:

> *Ms B said; "There were body parts in a bag and all the body liquids were seeping out. There were hands on me in the dark as I tried to get the door open and the door was forced shut- the hands were like tentacles like octopuses or like alien they were bright green- no head"*

This was discussed and she associated the feeling with the move to video calling in the virtual consulting room; *Ms B said, "I am not keen to do video calls yet, but I am aware you have moved to this new virtual and want to be in on it with the other clients".* So she feels ambivalent about the intrusiveness and yet, not wanting to miss out. She then said, *"I do not know why you would think about going back face to face with clients. It is so risky for you and your house hold, having them in your house again. If you can work remotely why not just do that? That is perfectly fine- it is too risky.*

Considering that she was an NHS worker, at some possible risk herself, that was a very protective as well as projective thought, about keeping me safe, she also went on to indicate that the psychotherapy job is the worst to be in at the moment as psychotherapists are fielding all of the anxiety in society. This could be thought of as a projection of her own risk, and it is also about keeping the room and me in it a safe *Stage 4 Consulting Room-object + transference* and preserved. The following week Ms B managed, perhaps somehow by protecting me, to have her first video call session, after a brief practice that week which she discussed in this session:

> *Ms B said, "It is not just the session it is the journey to you and the room and the journey away- zoom seems very definite- the screen just goes blank, on the phone we say goodbye. I am alright, I am in the house anyway. I don't have to go anywhere I don't have a partner about to walk in at any minute. I don't have to make my way home. I pictured I was going to sit up at the table as that is what people do on the TV- sit at a table – but I am too tired to sit it up, I was really tense last week about what it would be like- would it be worrying, stressful about being seem? what does everyone else do? where do they sit? Then this week I am not worried at all, I just thought oh. It doesn't matter so I am in my nighty. I remember the walk to the room, it was cosmic- wild- the foxes were in street sometimes. Walking to you and away from yours is part of the process, part of the event, with zoom it is off- bang! It's a shock- walking to and from is in control- going and coming*
>
> *I said, "and saying goodbye and walking down the path"*
>
> *She then said, "Yes, I would prefer if I switched it off first and then it won't feel like a shock to feel left."*

Having the video call session was a very big step to me seeing into her flat and her in her flat, for that to feel safe, and to make something good and containing of it, and for me to somehow witness something of the creation of it, this added a totally new spatialised dimension to the work, on video call. In that first video call/virtual session, I had a good view of the wallpaper that got damaged by the man and carefully fixed by Ms B. This is reminiscent of the image (Fig. 3.2 page 80) for *Stage 2 – Room object* based on Ms B's relationship with the walls which she used to hug, like Mums skin. She managed to repair the wallpaper herself, working towards a *Stage 5 – original Room-object + Consulting room-object + me in the transference* all in the new room. By the following session, she had gained confidence with the opportunities of the medium. She sat in the same spot with the wallpaper behind her (see Fig. 6.5 where the figure looks at the therapist in the screen who has the same vertical wallpaper from painting Fig. 3.2 behind).

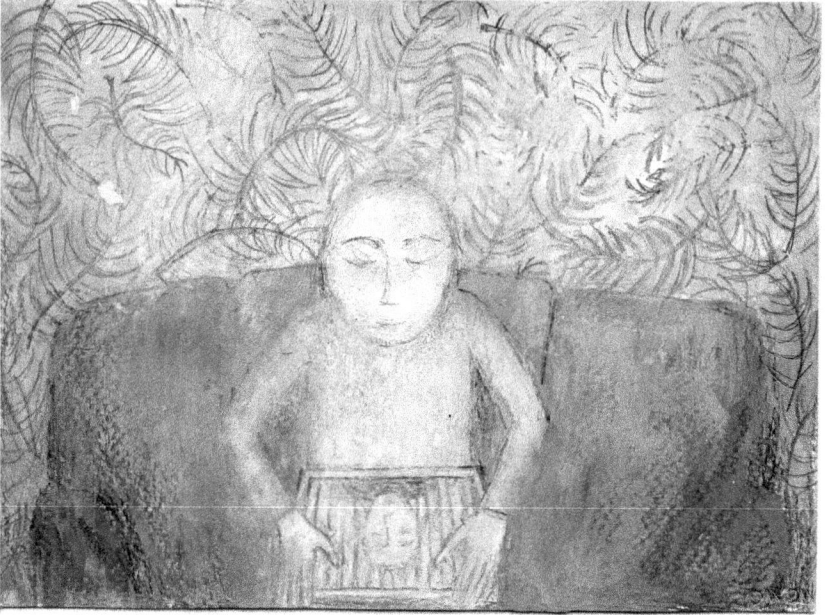

Figure 6.5 Re-projected Room-object and Matrix Stage 5; Wall paper and skin in the virtual Consulting Room. Drawing by D. Wright.

Ms B talked about her annual leave and how she want to do things in the house, she then showed me her sofa and said, "I am going for a theme of mustard and black and white", and she showed me the table she wants to set up as a desk on and talked about a new duvet cover and sheet sets. "I have not bought stuff like that for ages."

She then showed me clothes that she had bought that all seemed like a new and novel opportunity, that suddenly seemed quite exciting rather than worrying about how to do it, or me seeing into the room feeling intrusive. She had the next session tucked up in bed, 'with the electric blanket on', which not only brings the safety to the bedroom, where previously here the workman had 'removed the bulb' it also had the effect of feeling like telling a bedtime story before bed and tucked up to go to sleep, like a very safe and not-bad Room-object scenario.

She said, 'I want to live in place where I feels safe, where I no longer feel frightened and jump. I do feel safer now in this flat that was the point of the flat, I just want to feel safe in my own home- I hope to achieve that. I often still do not feel safe especially in the living room- we talked about the living room feeling un safe".

This was a very important thing for her to be able to think about and it seemed that if we have not had a situation where I had been able to see the space of her flat and feel comfortable with me seeing it, she would not have been able to think about her own discomfort in the way she had.

The Last Session Before the Christmas Break (9 Months After the Virtual Consulting Room Move)

Since Ms B had moved to mainly phone sessions two years previously, she had always come to the consulting room for her last session before the Christmas break. This kept the space of 'Christmas' safe by bringing items bought for it from the shop near my house into the consulting room, to be looked at, thought about together, or left in their bag (either way, made good), and then taken home to have over the break to keep 'Christmas' safe and the break good. During lockdown this could not happen.

Ms B said, " hello"

I said, "Oh you are in the kitchen"

She said, "Oh yes, well it is during the day I am in my living room".

I asked her about her table position, as I was not sure where it was in relation to the kitchen. She moved the lap top around and showed me the wall one side then the other. She then discussed the kitchen – showed me the shelves, the spice racks- the glass containers and their labels, the bread bin, the scales, the pink bin for waste food. She said, "The wall paper on the other wall seemed like it might be cold- it has taken me a long time to get to know this flat- at first I really did not understand the space – it has taken me a long time to get to know the space – it really has- I didn't have clue when I first came here- I tried all sort of things- I did not know what worked. It takes a long time to really get to know a space and what it right for it- you have to try lot of things first. Maybe it is just me – I am fussy and need to get it right."

I said. " it feels like it is a project that you are still working on now, it is an on-going project – a work in progress, that you now feel you have been making some headway with, it feels like you are getting to a place you are happy with now"

Ms B said, "Yes, well with the wallpaper it seemed cold then I balanced it up with this baby pink paint here to make it warmer", she shows me the wall, "and then I brought that through in the colour of the accessories in the kitchen- the cabinets are mushroom – so you have to be careful to use muted colours -so it is like – it needs to be pastels"

Then after showing the wall paper and wall image, she showed the pink wall- the side board- solid wood- with plants and tinsel on it.

She said, "Oh I put that up this morning- I went to the shops this morning to get the Christmas food and then came back and put up the Christmas decorations, I don't feel Christmassy thought yet..." She talked about the Christmas tree showing it, and the table it was on. Then talked about the shops and food. "For Christmas day I am doing garlic bread myself as there were no garlic bread slices." Ms B showed the bread like a cooking show – demonstrated cutting it- she showed me her magic mixer and explained you can put in the butter and garlic and herbs and the spread it and then put it in the freezer. She will make Walldorf salad roast parsnips and salad- she showed me the lettuce.

At the end of session, I said, "so it seems that you have got your shopping, like you normally do before you come, put up your decorations and now you have had your pre-Christmas session".

Ms B said, "yes I can start to feel Christmassy now."

Having the 'pre-Christmas session' in the virtual consulting room created a whole spatialised aspect to the event with quite a lot of showing of things as if I was witnessing a trial run of the preparation, in particular the cooking part, it was the food, and the association of normally buying it and bring it to my room before having it, here buying it and showing it to me was sufficient to 'feel Christmassy' and safe.

Clinical Example: Mr H (Who had 2 Sessions in the Room Before the Virtual Consulting Room Move)

Mr H, mid-20s, has been working with me in Consulting room 3 for 2 sessions prior to the move to the virtual consulting room. Mr H's presenting problem was chronic depression which he describes as living with a "bag over my head", over a number of years that was almost completely debilitating to functioning at times. His self-care was poor and his eating was limited to very simple raw vegetables/salads or smoothies/liquid foods. Also, anxiety and OCD symptoms manifesting in stuck thinking, difficulty with containing thinking. In his early childhood, his parents argued constantly, and they split with he was 7, his mother leaving with him and his brother, to live in another house and he does not recall having space of his own, his early bedroom that he lost, or the room at his father's new house which at times shared with his brother. He cannot remember feeling like any space was his or felt comfortable or settled. He also had to look after his mother's house and slept in his mother's bed till 10. His mother was narcissistic and emotional, 'un-boundaried' needy and ineffectual as doing things, his father, a successful academic, was distant and unemotional, did not stop mum's needs impacting on Mr H once he was gone, whilst also disapproving and judging of things. He described me at one point as weaning him off his parents, to which he made a connection with his eating liquidised foods. "*I am trying to think about myself and my own identity as separate from my family- it is all new I feel very young".* He had a phantasy of living in a phantasy cottage in Wales from aged 14 which felt self-reliant. Mr H had had 2 sessions in the Physical Consulting room before the move to the Virtual Consulting room. His initial feeling about working in the Virtual Consulting room were "disappointment" and being "not happy". The difficulty at the beginning in the virtual consulting room was compounded by the Easter Break, in the last session before the break:

> Mr H said, "I don't know how you feel- I mean I am just in a room all day – looking at people on like- I mean – (he puts hands on his face and rally cries) it is what I do all day- just look at people through the screen, you must know I miss you working in the room... I mean ... it feel like I don't know if I can be seen – it is just through a screen ... Can you see me? I might seem fine ... I was wondering if you can see that I am not I am not right?- I feel terrible."

> I said, "I can see and it might feel worrying that I can hold it in mind through the break"

He feels distant from the room and me and is worried about the break that contained the *Stage 4* transference elements, as well as the virtual consulting room object, which would be *Stage 5*. But perhaps, as his own mother was so intrusive and demanding and he lacked a sense of own space, he felt that the physical space of the consulting room needed to provide that space, he felt forced out of it by me (as mother) and then felt unseen and without a room object or mother's positive attention and regard. First, the room was lost in the virtual move, then me in the break – so sensory *Stage 1 – primary spatialisation*, allowed for spontaneous abandoned feeling similar to that which Mr C had in the original room move in Chapter 4. Being alone in the space means keeping intruding feelings at bay himself. Fig. 6.6, shows this 'bad' Virtual consulting Room-object, that easily gets intruded on, that does not feel his, (feels isolated in parts) loses the good Consulting room-object into which he put elements of the original good *Stage 1 Room-object* that he had to leave when his parents split but can hardly remember as did not have it long enough. Two months after the Virtual Room-move, Mr H was still considering this;

> Mr H said, "If we were in the room you would be able to see the whole me, I think you could see more of me, like see me all over so you could

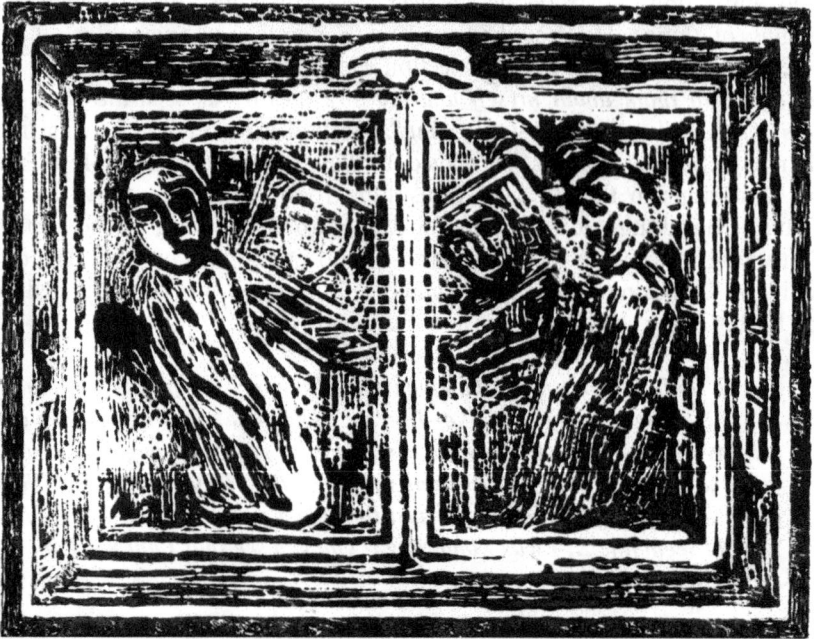

Figure 6.6 The Bad Consulting Room-object- Virtual Consulting room space IV. Lino Cut by D. Wright.

observe all of my hand movements and my feet movements. I think in the room I would not be able to gaze at you so long when you are talking like today. I was looking at you for 10 minutes- I wouldn't be able to do that"

It is interesting that he used the word gaze, as that is a word that might be associated with babies 'gazing' at their mother's whilst feeding, as in a 'Mirrored'(Winnicott, 2002) experience. Mr H is suggesting an unexpected benefit of the Virtual Consulting room, where he feels he can gaze uninterrupted, contradicting Kate Murphy's suggestion that; 'Authentic expressions of emotion [...] all but disappear on pixelated video [...] it also plays havoc with our ability to mirror.' (Murphy, 2020) Alessandra Lemma writes, 'The most readily available and deployed mirror in the twenty-first century that had supplanted all others is the *black mirror*. This is the one you will find on virtually every desk, in every home, and in the palm of every hand: the cold, shiny screen of a monitor, tablet or phone. (Lemma, 2017, p. 47). So, although we could say that Figs. 6.1, 6.2, and 6.3 all contain mirroring elements in a virtual setting where there is a double mirroring via the screen- the *'black mirror'* as Lemma calls it and, especially at the beginning of working in the Virtual consulting room, I was very conscious to ensure that the patients had a mirroring experience by my ensuring that I was looking at the camera and checking their expressions. Mr H is talking about something slightly different as well though. He is concerned about being seen entirely, so he often sat back from the camera screen, so that I can see him as a whole. This is shown in Fig. 6.7, in which he is hugged up against the walls of his room (almost held by the walls), where there is a feeling of being far away, isolation, and aloneness and yet also a gaze that he report he would never normally have done and an expectation of being gazed at. This feels like a very early experience of feeding and gazing but set up to feel better by him than his early intruded on experiences. The distance is also safe in another way.

Sometimes he moved around the room to get a comfortable space, whilst holding his laptop, which feels similar to what Shulman and Saroff (2020) discuss as feeling like a transitional object when the device is carried around, whilst they are inside it. This can sometimes result in Mr H taking up a position bundled up on the floor with blankets (in particular during the winter months) with the laptop very close up (as shown in Fig. 6.8). Gillian Issacs Russel writes, similarly to Murphy and Lemma, 'When we use technology, whether a computer or a phone, the loss of many subtle non-verbal cues means that we have to work so much harder to perceive the whole communication. When working face-to-face on screen, the view of the face without the whole body is closer than with in-person connection and distracting.'

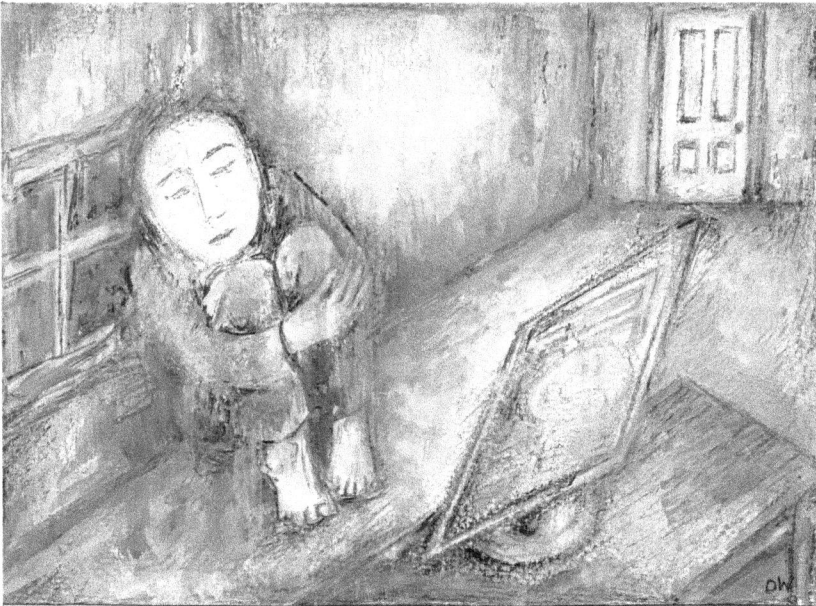

Figure 6.7 Far Away- The Virtual Consulting room space IV. Painting by D. Wright.

(Issacs Russell, 2020, p. 367). Here she is talking about an unusual closeness facially. Fig. 6.8 shows this very close-up experience. Mr H is experimenting with the space of close and distant, looked at and being looking at. This would a combination of a good *Stage 2 Room-object*, a good Stage 3 Consulting Room-object and a good Stage 4 – Consulting Room-object + transference. With gazing and close proximity of face and head and so on, closer up view – a lot of look and closeness and distance. But also safe as there is no possibility of physical intrusion. However, in a session 9 months after the move during this winter period, he talked about his need to repeatedly clean his room and the windows checking everything for dust before sitting down, he was expressing an unsafeness in his room that he also felt in my room, showing the unsafeness around in the virtual consulting room too:

> *Mr H said, "I Don't like the books behind you it really bothers me, they might be gathering dust. Mum's house is very dusty and there are papers and magazines with dust on them and broken drawers in the bedroom and can't be fixed and have tried to fix them. I would like you to put journals or whatever they are and books away in drawers or something or in a book case with doors the you would not get all the dust – it is bad for you."*

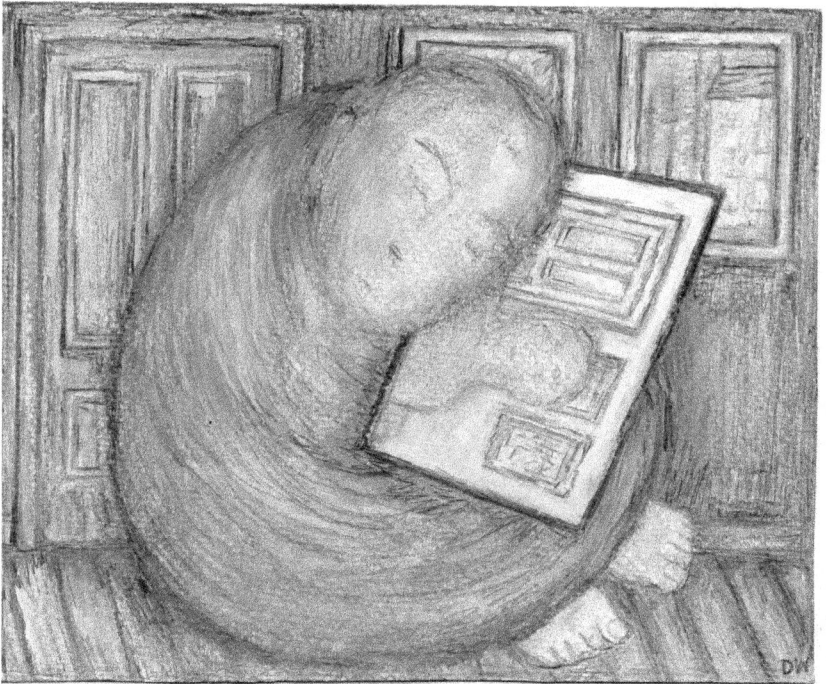

Figure 6.8 Close Together – The Virtual Consulting room space V. Painting by D. Wright.

We could say that this is a bad *Stage 3 Consulting Room- object* as well as *Stage 4* including the transference reflecting Mother's house where she and the house feel toxic, depressed, and unfunctional. He is worried that I will be infected by the consulting room – it could be dangerous. He then went on to discuss his difficulty with doing laundry and drying it in his flat, it is hard to get his sheets washed. As he discusses this, I am aware of feeling like a witness to a difficult and problematic space – looking into the whole scene, but my seeing it with him, like Ms F and Ms B seems to have importance in the thinking about it in a very immediate way. Mr H moves about in the space at times or situated himself in different past do the room, and in different positions, floor, bean bag, chair, and so on, to suit his mood spatially which we discuss. In a subsequent session, he had the session from sitting on the floor surrounded by his laundry racks, which I asked him about and he realised was a way of showing me (spatially) that he had been able to do his laundry. *He said "I had a good weekend for the first time in years – e just pottered around but it felt good, he cleaned the flat on the Saturday instead of not being able to do"* His own space is beginning to become less toxic to be in, and less bad *Room-object*.

A year after the room move, he had for the first time, a memory of his early life that contained happy elements, (a good *Room-object* space as opposed to the bad *Room-object* where he was worried about the books and journals behind me being covered in dust and infecting me like his mother's house does to him):

> *Mr H said, "I had a memory of my parent's old house when I was really young when I look at old videos of myself of when I was young I looked happy – it was chaotic- there was an assortment of odd chairs in the garden, it was very middle class, there were a lot of people around- I can remember running in and out of the garden, there was stuff everywhere it was messy and chaotic, things, art work, good furniture, but he thinks there was happy times."*

He thought about how, when his parents split when Mr H was around 8, he went from being relatively carefree in this memory running around with not much attention on him, to after the spit having a lot of attention from his mother that felt intrusive/looking after his mother's needs. In the earlier memory, even though his parents were in conflict, he had some sense of space to run around in this environment, that he suddenly had a happy memory of. He then had an important realisation; that he feels like he has never had a thought that was just his, not intruded on, this was a very important thing for him to consider, what it would actually be like to have his own thoughts, not for someone else.

In the next session, he said that he had put an offer in to buy a flat. He was excited to show a picture of the flat on 'screen share', and talked about feeling happy that it is his choice for only him. Thinking about the good and bad *Room-objects*, the closeness, intrusion, and distance, the Virtual Consulting room enabling additional spatialised elements, that would not have happened in the physical consulting room enabling to creation of the *Stage 5* space.

Clinical Examples: Mr J (All Work was in the Virtual Consulting Room)

Mr J, aged 30, began working with me in the virtual consulting room 2 months after the move to the virtual consulting room. So, Mr J had never been in the physical space of the consulting room, but much like Mr E, beginning work with me after the room move to room '3' (Chapters 4 and 5) they both arrived at the new room with no thought of the other room as they had never been in it. Mr J got straight into the work without considering the physical room that we moved from or the surroundings, as Ms F and Ms G and Mr H did. So, although Mr J did notice my background surroundings, when, on session 2 he remarked, "Ah you have been moving your office", he noticed that I had moved things in my background, (from Consulting room '3' to create a more familiar background for everyone), Mr J had no particular feeling about it. Mr J's presenting problem was unhappiness relating to difficulties with the ending of his marriage. This led him to binge drinking alone and going through a ritual of watching 'The Lion King' and crying. He felt that this was an emotional release and it made him think of his father, who he wanted to us think about, and who had passed away. Mr J felt that he had never got to know him. When his mother brought, he and his siblings to England, when he was 7, his father had stayed in Pakistan and he only saw him in the holidays. His father could also not help him deal with his mother's bipolar disorder. He can remember that his mother did not pay much attention to him *"she was very depressed she didn't notice me"*, when she was subdued and depressed, sleeping a lot, or when she had manic phases of talking angrily sometimes about his dad. He only vaguely remembered his house in Pakistan. In England, they lived in his cousin's house, he thinks that he may have shared bedrooms with his brother – he can't remember the room or any things that he had. Mr J remembers being bullied at primary school as he feels he was overweight as he always ate the **"wrong type of food"** he did not feel cared for. He is aware that he has compensated for that in his adult life but taking good care of what he looks like, clothes, exercise, gym, and so on. When he was 13, they moved house to a bigger house, owned by his older sister, and he had his own box room. He had lived in the house ever since, and it was his first *Stage 2 Room-object* space. When he and his wife got married, they bought the house from his older sister and the family home became his. At the breakdown of his marriage, he was left living in it and did not know what to do. He did not want to sell it as it was his first *Stage 2 Room-object space*, so he was deciding whether to buy out his wife's share of the house so he could keep it.

Thinking about the significance of the house and showing me it – the kitchen and dining area, with the lap top- was an important part of the work at the beginning. In the sessions, Mr J established his relationship with the house and how he felt about it so he could try moving from it. ***He said, "Can a house contain Karma? Bad memories might get stuck in the house- they might infect a new relationship, if I changed the lay-out of the furniture that might help"***. He was trying to work out if the space was a good object space – good enough to survive what had happened and if he can save it and transform its meaning as he wants to keep it a good *Stage 2 Room-object* space. This contrast with earlier bad objects space difficulties with mother and later with his wife. He wanted to begin a new relationship with someone at his work and wondered if that will be good or get affected, if he can leave the house, there are bad memories but it is his first memorable good *Stage 1 Room-object* space room as well. A few months after beginning the work and talking about the house and its meaning, Mr J said that he has decided to move out and give his ex-wife 50% of the proceeds as that is what she had wanted. He said, *"there are a lot of bad memories in the house now and things feel very bad here sometimes"*. Six months later Mr J had moved away from the family home and was living in a new flat in the area that he had phantasies about *"getting away"* to and separating from his family and becoming independent from them and from mother. *He said that it is, "a relief to live away from the family where everyone is around the corner, and to feel some space and separation."*

Although he had also begun a new relationship, he is careful to live in a separate space to her so they can get to know each other and to be reassured that she is not like his mother as well as try living on his own for the first time which he felt was important. It was not easy for him, he said it is, *"difficult to get to know my new girlfriend"* as they do not see much of each other. He was having the session in the living room of his new rented flat with the cardboard Box, from his new TV sitting across his background like he is displaced and unsettled which was different to the homely domestic kitchen scene of the home he left. He was doubting about his ability to re-create a better *Stage 2 Room-object* space anywhere else. Meanwhile, I was wondering about his creating a *Stage 5* space for the sessions when he has never been in the consulting room to introject it and re-spatialise it there. He managed it though.

2 Months Later in the First Session After the Christmas Break

Mr J said, "I am is having the session in the car today as I had to come in for work and in the office I am not sure people cannot perhaps hear and the walls are very thin- I can hear in there ... I am in the car anyway then I can go in. The break was very difficult this year. Normally I have time with my family over Christmas and new year- I spend time with them and I just didn't. I thought that when I moved to here that I would spend more time with my girlfriend, I just haven't, I feels very alone I feel very depressed".

He looks out of the car - although it was the middle of the day, it was quite dark. He said "the cold weather is very depressing. You know- I was drinking Brandy for about 4 days out of the break- the time between Christmas and new year is the worst- I was thinking in the lock down, I was alright because I still exercise, I was out in the garden at the park and so on. So, I decided that I need to exercise more as it is good for me- also I was eating rubbish really and I put on quite a bit of weight before Christmas and it is a shame because I lost it all when I was in the house in the summer. It happened before I moved here ..."

I said, "it has been hard as we have had our break and you left the house and everything is new"

This is *Stage 4 – Consulting-room object + transference* but he also had a *Stage 1 Primal spatialisation* feeling of being displaced from everything, feeling of home, *Stage 2 Room-object*, the Virtual consulting Room-object, and me in the break.

Mr J said, "when I moved here, I had not expected to be alone so much, but being alone should not be a big deal- I needs to be comfortable with it and not frightened."

I said, "Your original phantasy about moving "away" was related to independent thinking and separation from family, it does not feel very independent, it feels difficult".

He said, "Yes, it's not as easy as it seems, I did expect her to be there... but I can see that it would be a good thing to be comfortable with being alone ... it is funny as my wife was there all the time and never left me alone and I did not like that."

I said, "There is something else here – the two locations and women seem like two sides to mum- the manic, intrusive, non-stop talking side and the withdrawing depressed side - the side that ignored you, neglecting your needs."

Mr J said, "Oh yes I can't win there- but I need to be comfortable being alone though."

On the following session he said, "I am not so lonely now, my girlfriend has a new cat, he sits on my knee-he is black cat, I like that. I was very frightened to move away to this flat-even though it is only up the road really not far."

Things feel more integrated here and less 'polarised' in terms of locations and his feelings.

Conclusions

In The Virtual consulting room, patients have had to be creative in their spatialising outside the consulting room space. As Lemma writes; 'technological developments are 'developments' in the sense that they have created opportunities for extending learning and creativity and they may be used by some individuals to assist developmental processes' (Lemma, 2015, p. 570). This chapter has looked at the creative use of the Virtual Consulting-room space involving 'Screen sharing 'in the example of Mr A in Chapter 1, the use of email as an extension of the room space on the screen and in the mind with Ms G, and a conceptualisation of the 'Virtual Consulting-room spaces' as an overarching conceptual room, in the case of Ms F, which can be seen as existing in the therapist and patient's mind. We have also looked at the use of the spatial array of location 'good' and 'bad', around the Virtual consulting room where patients have shown room spaces, gardens, and objects that they have made, and things that they have done to rooms to create the *Stage 5 Consulting Room-object + Transference, outside the Consulting room.* This has constituted a large part of the work, in some cases including those who had barely or not been in the physical consult room space, but for whom the Virtual space of the consulting room can also be seen to have contributed significantly to the patient's therapeutic experience.

Figure References

Figure 6.1: On-line working in room spaces. Painting by D. Wright.

Figure 6.2: The Virtual Consulting room space I. Drawing by D. Wright.

Figure 6.3: Room-object Spatial Matrix: Stage 5: The Virtual Consulting Room-object + Transference, outside the Consulting room. Drawing by D. Wright.

Figure 6.4: Home from Home; The Virtual Consulting room space III. Drawing by D. Wright.

Figure 6.5: Re-projected Room-object and Matrix Stage 5; Wall paper and skin in the virtual Consulting Room. Drawing by D. Wright.

Figure 6.6: The Bad Consulting Room-object- Virtual Consulting room space IV. Lino Cut by D. Wright.

Figure 6.7: Far Away- The Virtual Consulting room space IV. Painting by D. Wright.

Figure 6.8: Close Together – The Virtual Consulting room space V. Painting by D. Wright.

References

Aryan, A. (2019) Psychoanalytic process in Cyber-technology (pp. 65–89) *Psychoanalysis Online 4: Teleanalytic Practice, Teaching and Clinical Research.* Editor: Jill Savege Scharff). London & New York, Routledge.

Bate J., and Malberg, N. (2020) Containing the Anxieties of Children, Parents and Families from a Distance During the Coronavirus Pandemic. *Journal of Contemporary Psychotherapy.* 50:285–294. Published online: 14 July 2020, 10.1007/ s10879-020-09466-4 © Springer Science+Business Media, LLC, part of Springer Nature 2020.

Bonaminio, V. (2010) Psychoanalysis and virtual reality. *International Journal of Psychoanalytical Panel report,* 91:985–988.

Carlino, R. (2010) *Distance psychoanalysis.* London: Karnac.

Dini, K. (2009) Internet interaction: The effects on patient's lives and analytic process. *JAPA,* 57:979–988.

Ermann, M. (2004) On medial identity. *International Forum of Psychoanalysis,* 13: 275–283.

Fiorentini, G. (2012) Laanalisi via Internet: variazioni di setting e dinamiche transferali-controtransferali. *Rivista di Psicoanalisi,* 58(1):29–45.

Issacs Russell, G. (2015) *Screen Relations: The Limits of Computer-mediated Psychoanalysis and Psychotherapy.* London: Karnac.

Issacs Russell G. (2020) Remote Working During the Pandemic: A Q&A with Gillian Isaacs Russell Questions from the Editor and Editorial Board of the BJP. *British Journal of Psychotherapy.* 36, 3 (2020) 364–374 John Wiley & Sons Ltd

Kachele, H. (2019) Case Study Research A Psychotherapeutic Relationship established by email (pp. 49–59). In: *Psychoanalysis Online 4: Teleanalytic Practice, Teaching and Clinical Research.* Editor: Jill Savege Scharff). London & New York, Routledge.

Kilborne, B. (2011) Personal communication with Alessandra Lemma as referred to in Lemma A. (2015). *International Journal of Psycho-Analysis,* 96(3): 569–582.

Leader, C. (2021) 'LOCKED DOWN'; Reflections from the consulting room during the Covid-19 pandemic. *New Associations British Psychoanalytic Council* Issue 34 Summer 2021 London: British Psychoanalytic Council.

Lemma, A. & Caparrotta, L., editors (2014) Psychoanalysis in the technoculture era. London: Routledge.

Lemma, A. (2015) Psychoanalysis in Times of Technoculture: Some Reflections on the Fate of the Body in Virtual Space (2015). *International Journal of Psycho-Analysis.* 96(3):569–582.

Lemma, A. (2017) *The Digital Age on the Couch Psychoanalytic practice and New Media*. London & New York, Routledge

Lingiardi, V. (2008) Playing with unreality: Transference and computer. *The International Journal of Psychoanalysis*, 89: 111–126.

Manguel, L. (2019) *Psychoanalysis Online 4: Teleanalytic Practice, Teaching and Clinical Research*. (pp. 90–108) Editor: Jill Savege Scharff). London & New York: Routledge.

Murphy, K. (2020) Why Zoom Is Terrible There's a reason video apps make you feel awkward and unfulfilled. *The New York Times Sunday Review* https://www.nytimes.com/2020/04/29/Sunday-review/zoom-video-conference.html

Shulman Y. & Saroff A. "Imagination for Two" Child Psychotherapy during Coronavirus Outbreak: Building a Space for Play When Space Collapses, *Journal of Infant, Child, and Adolescent Psychotherapy*, ISSN: (Print) (Online) Journal homepage: https://www.tandfonline.com/loi/hicp2 Routledge

Vincent, C., Barnett, M., Killpack, L., Sehgal, A., Swinden, P. (2017) Advancing Telecommunication Technology and its Impact on Psychotherapy in Private Practice. *British Journal of Psychotherapy*. 33, 1, 63–76.

Winnicott, D. W. (2002 [1967]) Mirror-role of Mother and Family in Child Development. [First published 1967] *Playing and Reality*. London: Routledge. (1971, reprinted 2002), pp. 111–118.

Chapter 7

Beyond the Consulting Room; Psychosocial Applications of the Room-object Spatial Matrix to E.M. Forster's Post-colonial, Capitalist, Pre Neo-liberal, Queer, and Virtual Rooms and Spaces of his Novels

In this chapter, I will now apply the formulation of Room-object Spatial Matrix within a broader psychosocial set of contexts by utilising it to examine and consider Edward Morgan Foster's spaces and rooms in his novels. In so doing, I will also consider both the social themes he explored in his novels and the rooms and spaces within them and how applying the Room-object spatial Matrix can bring out psychosocial thinking on these themes and spaces allowing for an additional layer of thinking. These themes include post-colonial room spaces, capitalist room spaces (pre-neoliberal), as well as religious, class-based and queer room spaces within the spatial array of Forster's locations and rooms places as he formulated them. According to Andre Green 'Psychoanalytic theory has only one source, or at least an inescapable main source – the experience of what happens in the consulting room between the patient and the analyst' (Kohon, 1999, p. 29). I am here taking my formulation from the consulting room and applying it in a psychosocial context to Forster's works; 'A Passage to India', 'Howards End', 'A Room with a View', 'Maurice', and 'The Machine Stops' to both exemplify the matrix positions and to bring out further thinking on post-colonial rooms and Forster's spatial political elements. Massey writes that;

> it is part of my argument, not just that the spatial is political [...] but rather that thinking the spatial in a particular way can shake up the manner in which certain political questions are formulated, can contribute to political arguments already under way, and – most deeply – can be an essential element in the imaginative structure which enables in the first place an opening up to the very sphere of the political.
>
> (Massey, 2005, pp. 9–10)

I discussed spatialisation (Wright 2019) in the political realm, in relation to the fomenting of political violence. Here I am not only looking at the political in relation to my conceptualising of spatialisation, but I am also

DOI: 10.4324/9781003188117-7

utilising my formulation of the Room-object Spatial Matrix to analyse Forster's novels that afford a language describing a range of political expressions, in themselves spatial, and room based. This concerns people's relationships to the interiors of rooms, spaces, houses, streets, cities, and countryside, including colonial, post-colonial, capitalist (pre-neoliberal), and queer perspective spaces, often, we can also think of as expressions of stages on the Room-object Spatial Matrix, which I shall utilise to access and understand some of Forster's meanings and therefore aspects of the wider political and social issues on which he comments on spatially. This is turn will demonstrate and exemplify a psychosocial usage for the Room-object Spatial Matrix in a wider context to the Consulting room.

A Passage to India; Foster's Pre-Colonial, Colonial, and Post-colonial Spaces

For Deniz Kandiyoti; 'Within the field of postcolonial studies itself, Moore-Gilbert (1997) points to the divide between "post-colonial criticism," which has much earlier antecedents in the writings of those involved in anti-colonial struggles, and "post-colonial theory," which distinguishes itself from the former by the incorporation of methodological paradigms derived from contemporary European cultural theories into discussions of colonial systems of representation and cultural production (Kandiyoti, 2002, p. 279). And for Helen Gilbert and Joanne Tompkins 'post-colonialism is […]an engagement with, and contestation of, colonialism's discourses, power structures, and social hierarchies' (Gilbert & Tompkins, 1996, p.8). Foster was a post-colonial critic, in fact, 'A Passage to India', charts the end of the time of the British Raj and the breakdown of the colonial community. Oliver Stallybrass writes; 'A passage to India unquestioningly gave […] "vivid dramatic evidence to justify the direction of a swing that had already begun […] which enabled the British people to leave India"' (Forster, 1985[1924], pp. 21–22). However, Forster is also one of the first post-colonial writers, and one of the first to write from the perspective of characters from those colonised countries.

A Passage to India centres around the fictional community of Chandrapur where Mrs Moore, the mother of Ronny Heaslop (the local Magistrate), and Miss Adela Quested (Ronny's fiancé to be) arrive in Chandrapur and see the colonial community through fresh eyes. Mrs Moore is shocked at the change in her son and the way the community operates and Adela doubts whether she can marry him. Both women want to see the 'real India' (Forster, 1985[1924], p. 47). Forster shows these changes that happen to colonials that Mrs Moore and Adela are shocked by, in a conversation between Dr Aziz and his friends, where Dr Aziz explains to them that when Mr Turton (who we see in the novel along with his wife, as behaving in a particularly racist manor) first came out to India, that he was friendly with Dr Aziz. Dr Aziz talked humorously about getting lifts in Mt Turton's carriage and being shown his stamp collection. He concludes though that all Englishmen are the same and within 2 years they will have conformed to the colonial communities' attitudes and thinking. As Franz Fanon writes, 'The settler owes the fact of his very existence, that is to say, his property, to the colonial system' (Fanon, 1963[1961], p. 36) and '[i]n the colonial countries [...] the policeman and the soldier, by their immediate presence and their frequent and direct action maintain contact with the native and advise him by means of rifle butts [...] not to budge.' (Fanon, 1963[1961], p. 38). Foster writes of the colonial community allowing for the public school attitude to flourish in a way that it could not in England. Adela is envious when she discovers that Mrs Moor has seen the 'real India' beyond 'the club', in the ruined mosque (see Fig. 7.1) where she has a chance encounter with Dr Aziz. Foster writes

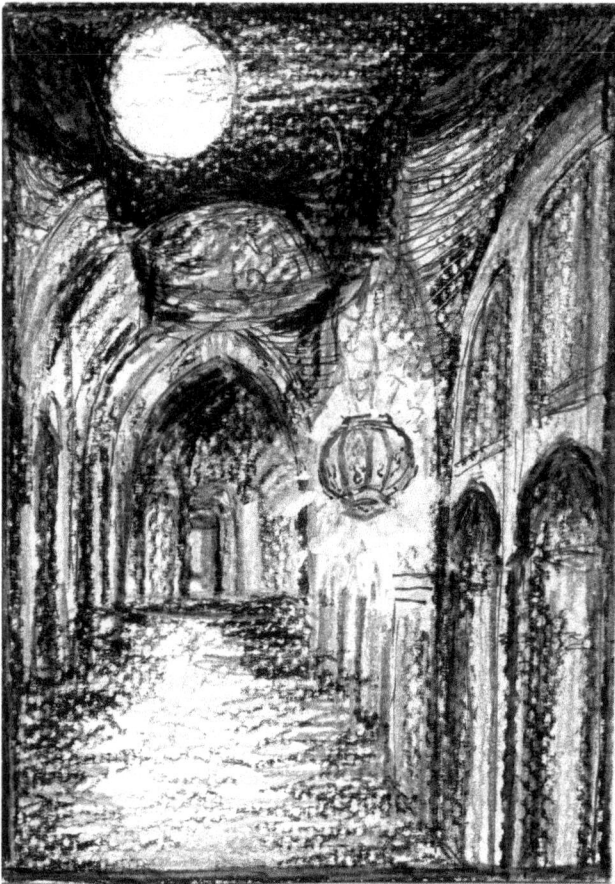

Figure 7.1 The Ruined Mosque. Drawing by D. Wright.

that when Aziz entered the ruined Mosque with its three arcades illuminated by a hanging lamp and by the moonlight of the full moon, he looked at the 99 names of God in the frieze, which stood out in black and he thought about Islam that he felt was an attitude to life both exquisite and durable. Dr Aziz felt that his body and his thoughts found their home not only in Islam, but he felt aware of all of that in the space of the ruined Mosque. As a religious building, we would expect it to contain transferential elements, like *Stage 3* of the matrix, where elements have been re-projected, re-spatialised. For Aziz, there is a re-spatialising of 'home'. However, as the Mosque is ruined, Forster represents it containing Stage 1 primal, pre-transferential elements, as nature has encroached on it and it is lit both by a lamp and by the moon. Mrs Moore takes off her shoes to enter saying that she feels that God is there in the ruined Mosque. She wants to join in with this spatialising but hints at the mysterious primal aspects. Aziz and Mrs Moore shared this primal experience at that moment and Aziz comments to Mrs Moore that as both of their spouses have died, they are therefore in the same box. This is an interesting space – is it like a coffin, certainly it is restrictive – both in terms of their grief but also the constrains from their societal positions across the colonial divide. However, the important thing is they are both in it together – in the ruined mosque space and the 'box' which is like a room and in this case a de-colonialised or post/beyond-colonial transcendent space of commonality of human experience. The *Stage 1 Primal spatialising* experience is shown to enabled them to be experientially out of their normal society roles in that moment. After the event, however, 'Colonialism', in the society around them, attempts to trample over the experience. Ronny talks about Dr Aziz to his mother, saying that he wishes that she had pointed Dr Aziz out as him as he can't think who he is. However, when Mrs Moore explains to Ronny that she cannot point Dr Aziz out to him in the club as Dr Aziz is not allowed in Ronny is shocked that she is was talking to a local Indian man, that he calls a 'native' whilst Miss Quested thinks it is magnificent and exclaims that whilst they talk about seeing the 'real India', Mrs Moore had just gone ahead and been seeing it and it seems so natural to Mrs Moore to have real experiences – not just talk about having them, that she even forgotten to let them know. Ronny, however, was angry that he could not influence his mother or that she would not capitulate to the colonial community thinking. He feels that Mrs Moore is influencing Adela to think uncolonially, which will mean it takes longer for Adela to fit in with the community or even that she will not want to marry Ronny and settle there at all.

The 'club' being the epicentre of all the colonial spaces, will not allow Aziz in, it is the space that defines the divide physically. Fanon writes; 'The zone where the natives live is not complementary to the zone inhabited by the settlers. The two zones are opposed, but not in the service of a higher unity. [...] they both follow the principle of reciprocal exclusivity.

(Fanon, 1963[1961], pp. 38–39). He is writing about two zones that we might think of as a splitting. I argue (2019) that the idea of splitting good and bad (Klein, 1946, p. 104) and projecting the bad out, can be linked with the ideas of sacred and profane, (Eliade, 1959), as discussed in Chapter 1 (see page 11). Control does not only take place – or better, is not only placed – within people, but rather within anything in the environment, such as buildings, objects, and landscapes. Fakhry Davids write about this in terms of racism;

> It has long been known that racist frames of mind involve splitting and projective identification [...] A paranoid solution to intense anxiety, this makes us feel that we know where we are, which helps, and can further justify actions designed to make us feel better, [...] The effects of such polarization are powerful and pervasive since racist thought seeks to present itself as the true picture of reality, sweeping up all in its path as it imposes its agenda and seeks to buttress its views. In the process alternative views are portrayed as being in the camp of the enemy.
>
> (Davids, 2002, p. 362)

The space of the 'club' is preserved as a spatial manifestation of this 'splitness' by the colonial communities justified keeping them inside and 'ruling' by virtue of their being white and everyone else outside and ruled. Fanon wrote, 'This disintegrating of the personality, this splitting and dissolution, all this fulfils a primordial function in the organism of the colonial world.' (Fanon, 1963[1961], p. 58). Fanon is using the word primordial, to describe this mechanism, that Forster showed Dr Aziz and his friends discussing of what happens to the colonial after they arrive in the community and we could think of this relating to a *Stage 1 – Primal spatialising*, action that feel unsafe and does not work, so the defences need to keep being shored up in a wider psychosocial sense. This is backed up by the narrative of the entire colonial community that keeps the 'club' intact and their sense of selves held together by the spatialising action of keeping it that way. This is reminiscent of the journey between the safe consulting rooms for Mr D, as depicted in Chapter 5 (see page 114) where the space between was fraught with projected dangers, which keeps the space safe and splits off the fear that it might not be safe, as in the case of consulting room 2 in Chapter 4, which did not feel safe and was broken into, as well as the split off split-off anger at me about all the danger that the room moves posed (Chapters 4 and 5). This society-agreed splitting relating to the club space is very different from the experience in the Mosque that felt spontaneous and transcendental of this splitting through *Stage 1 – Primal Spatialising* sensory experience.

Jean-Paul Sartre wrote 'this imperious being, crazed by his absolute power and by the fear of losing it, no longer remembers clearly that he was once a man; he takes himself for a horsewhip or a gun; he has come to believe that the domestication of the "inferior races" will come about by the conditioning of their reflexes.' (Sartre, 1963, pp. 16–17). Fanon also observes, 'The settler makes history and is conscious of making it. And because he constantly refers to the history of his mother country, he clearly indicates that he himself is the extension of that mother country.' (Fanon, 1963[1961], p. 51) He is suggesting that the 'mother' country as a whole is introjected and re-spatialised into the colonial space that replaces a kind of mother which is enacted. As we have seen in Chapters 1 to 3, Wollheim writes about states of mind directed upon spatial things: 'that we attribute to the mind thoughts about people and scenes, which are three-dimensional' (Wollheim, 1969, p. 216) but that in delusional psychosis, 'it might be possible to characterize the varying stages of mental disturbance, or the stations on the path to psychosis, by the degree to which the patient conceives of the mind, supremely of his mind, as a place. (Wollheim, 1969, p. 217). So, the colonial is replacing a space for thinking and experiencing with the idea of a space and in so doing spatialising by force a delusional mother country with almost complete spatialisation. Foster writes that in Chandrapore, the Turtons behaved like gods, but soon when they retire to a suburban villa somewhere, they would not be able to behave like Gods and would die physically separated from the glory that the Chandrapore community afforded them. This gives us an indication of their increased personal investment in maintaining the spaces of the community being divided up and spatialised in this way, including 'the club' at the epicentre of their power structure. Their God like status, as a delusional state, is highlighted, in that when they return home, they will be nothing – their meaning is through the colonial system, their house, and all the spatialised elements of colonial life.

Mrs Moore, rails against this, saying that the English should be there to add something to the community not for what they can get out of it, but because India is part of the earth that we all share and that God has put human beings onto earth to be kind to each other and she warns that God is omnipresent everywhere including India, to witness human's unkindness and cruelty to fellow humans. The English arrived in India, and they (along with their intentions) become a spatialised colonial version of themselves, that conforms to the expectations of the local expat community as well as the wider colonial concept. Aime Cesaire writes that '[t]hey prove that colonization, I repeat, dehuman even the most civilized man; that colonial activity, colonial enterprise, colonial conquest, which is based on contempt for the native and justified by that contempt, inevitably tends to change him who undertakes it; that the colonizer, who in order to ease his conscience gets into the habit of seeing the other man as an animal accustoms himself to treating him like an animal, and tends objectively to transform himself into an animal. (Cesaire, 2000, p. 43).

Against this already delusory backdrop, Adela Quested and Mrs Moore accept an offer from Dr Aziz to go on a picnic in the Marbar hills (partly so he will not have to have them at his house, which he feels is inadequate, and due to his being a widower he feels it is uncared for). Adela accepts this invitation, excitedly seeing it as a great opportunity for adventure. Forster writes that she believes that Dr Aziz can unlock the India for her, through seeing him as somehow representing the country and that she placed Dr Aziz on an idealised pinnacle. For her, he initially transcends the colonial community as she idealises him, splitting off getting to know him as an individual, (which Mrs Moore had been doing) and in her ignorance she does not realise – that although there is some transcendence of the colonial room space in private spaces – Mrs Moore and Dr Aziz at the mosque, Mr Fielding and Dr Aziz in each other's bedrooms, these are all private meetings in room spaces that can transcend the colonial room space of the 'club'. The Marbar Cave space event (see Fig. 7.2), which

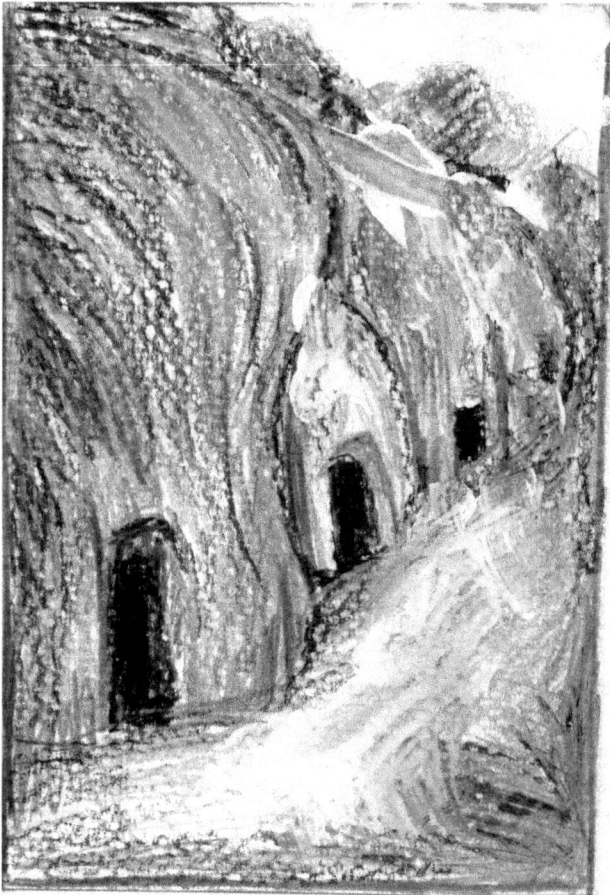

Figure 7.2 The Marbar Caves. Painting by D. Wright.

seems intimate and private between Dr Azis and Adela (where, as they climb up to the cave entrances they discuss relationships with some intimacy), in Adela's confusion then becomes public and therefore is viewed through the spatialised colonial lens and becomes a colonial space. Forster describes that as their elephant moved towards the Marbar hills, they seemed to move into an illusory space that was separate and cut off, from normal life, where sounds did not echo in the normal way and where thoughts were infected by illusion and did not develop. There was no thinking and the developing of an illusion – this fits with the primitive pre-thinking stage and in a different way the colonial elements, the phantasy about the 'real India' by Adela becomes shattered. Dr Aziz and Adela walk up to the cave entrances, and whilst Dr Aziz smoked a cigarette at the top, Adela wanders off into one of the caves entrances. The cave space is primal (*Stage 1*), pre-meaning, pre-transferential, and pre-colonial. Forster describes that for Adela, the echo in the caves seemed, in a way that would be impossible for her to describe, to undermine everything that she was familiar with and that she would associate with her life as she knew it to be. We do not know what actually happens to Adela in the cave but we know she impresses he own meaning upon it – she thinks, or the idea is put to her by the community that she has been attacked by Dr Aziz. Forster describes Dr Aziz's experience when he loses Adela after she enters one of the caves and his panic that he has lost her. As Dr Aziz looks for her in all of the caves, Forster describes the primalness of the caves as seeming to be like orifices that spawn more caves in an endless and disturbing closed circuit and trapping way, like the intrusive mother space that is discussed further on in this chapter in his novel 'Maurice' where Maurice's mother's house is also primally trapping and claustrophobic (whereas Maurice's therapists' consulting room seems to offer some potential space from that). The guide adds to this perception by explaining to Dr Aziz that a Marbar cave can only hear its own sounds. Here it seems to be saying that once in the cave, the projections onto the space almost seal off the inhabitant to all external projections - colonial, idealised, or otherwise and that there is something pre-verbal – pre-birth – womb-like shown in the orifices (see Fig. 7.2 showing 'orifices' of the cave entrances).

During the trial the Deputy Magistrate asks if the caves are Buddist or Jain; however, this is not clear, and it seems if pre-organised religion cannot seem to be impressed upon the caves by any pre-organised spatialised projection. Foster wrote later that the event in the cave could have been an illusion with sensory hallucinatory elements. In the trial, the delusion unravels and she seems enabled, through thinking about her indescribable experience in the cave, to be able to think about the reality without the colonial cultural spatialisation or her own confusion about how she feels about Ronny, the life there, or Dr Aziz, as she remembers that Dr Aziz was not in the cave with her.

Forster's reader is left to speculate about what she had experienced in the cave – the pre-verbal, pre-colonial, primal construct. At first, the cave trip seems to transcend the colonial spaces, for Adela. However, her idealising of Dr Aziz is muddled and breaks down, her unconscious feelings in the space are unfathomable, and as Fanon put it 'primordial', and she resorts to the colonial to contain this turning the cave into a colonial space. In the end, she enters the depressive position and allows the cave to return to a neutral pre- and post-colonial space transcendent of definition.

Howards End; Foster's Pre-neo-liberal Room Spaces, Bourgeois Literary and Artistic Room Spaces and the Primal Country Spaces

'Only connect', the phrase on the title page of Forster's book 'Howards End', relates to the families and the 'Howards End' house at the centre of the story, where families of very differing classes attempt to 'Connect' with each other and, in different ways, the house. Like the Marbar Caves, the house 'Howards End' (see Fig. 7.3, this drawing was based on the house that Forster grew up

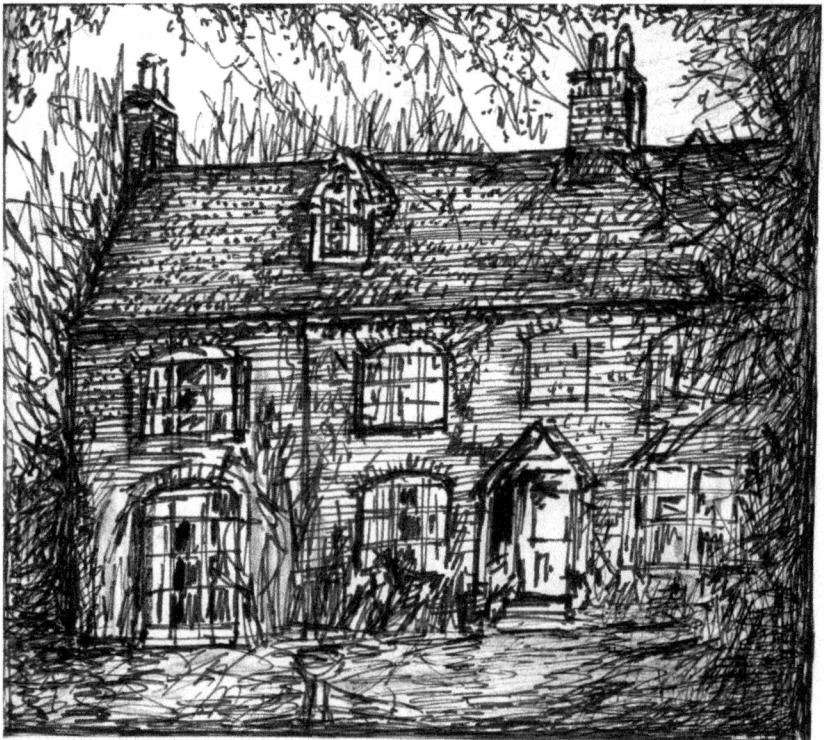

Figure 7.3 Howards End, Drawing by D. Wright.

in, which it is believed he based Howards End on) has *Stage 1 Primal Spatialisation* elements that seem to go beyond the Capitalist, Bourgeois, or working-class constructs that interplay through the characters. Like the Marbar Caves, the house seems neutral, transcendent, pre- or beyond neo-liberal thinking and concerns. The tree and the house seem 'Primordial' like the caves. Mrs Wilcox seems to be of the house and one with it and appears somewhat complacent to anything not concerning it. Forster describes that Mrs Wilcox does not belong to the current age with young people and motor cars, but to the house (Howards End) itself and the witching elm tree outside it. He described her as having instinctive wisdom connected to the house and to her ancestors that had inhabited it. Her own original *Stage 2 – Room-object* site is there and she is not interested in anything else (or re-spatialising this Room-object into any other space), stating it would kill her if she moved that and has no interest in the capitalist progress of the husband.

The Schlegel siblings are Bourgeois, artistic, and literary. Their central London terraced house is also a *Stage 2 Room-object* space for them, re-placing their parents, who died when they were young. Forster describes their old tasteful terraced house as sitting quietly and serenely behind the streets in front that had been developed into expensive modern London flats in which enormous entrance halls contained palms and concierges. Forster warns that the Schlegel's home, a peaceful town equivalency of Howards End, will not have the space to exist much longer as it is going to be taken away from them as it is due for development into flats as well. Forster de-scribes that the cost of land in London drives out the old and creates flats that go up into the sky but lack the connection to the land and the primal relationship to ancestors that Howards end represents. On discovering that the Schegel's home will be taken away from them and the space developed, Mrs Wilcox is horrified for them and says that Howards End was once nearly pulled down and that if it had been it would have killed her. She cannot function without being in her *Stage 2 Room-object* environment of Howards End and despite her staying in such a developed flat in London (representing capitalist progress with entrance halls with 'palms') – she cannot re-spatialise the Room-object space of Howards End into the flat in a *Stage 3* way. Forster comments on capitalist room space (original eighteenth Century 'Liberal' capitalism, pre- to the neo-liberal today but essentially the equivalent in room spaces) as bulldozing over the original spaces all over London. In a less salubrious area of London, where Leonard Bast lives, unlike the Capitalist Room spaces of the new flats Forster described, these working-class flats do not have 'palms' in the hallway. Leonard enters Block B of the flats and walks downstairs into what Forster humorously describes that 'house-agents' would call a semi-basement, but is actually a cellar. Forster describes the interior of the furnished flat, in detail, and that when the curtains are drawn, at night, that it could seem led worn and be made homely, but the lack of personal attachment to the furniture and objects in the space made it hard to fully what I am calling spatialise. There is something temporary, flimsy, and barely *Stage 3* about it. Forster observes that in this area too, although it is a working-class area, like everywhere else in London, it could disappear and be replaced with new higher flats, the vastness of which at present would have been unimaginable. Writing this in 1910, Forster was predicting the council flat building programmes of the 1950s onwards and questioning the concept of home, the individual connection to the land, and spatialising in spaces that can be removed by not having control over these room spaces.

Mr Wilcox represented this capitalist 'progress', on which Helen Schlegel commented that the Wilcox family seem like frauds, relating to things like newspapers, golf, cars, and other capitalist forms of middle-class pursuits, that masks emptiness and panic, as opposed to her form of middle-class existence that incorporated meaning through art, literature, and philanthropic ideals. Again, we have the idea that Capitalist spatialisation, like colonial spatialisation, is a splitting process to defend against 'emptiness'.

A Room with a View; Italy and the Church

'A Room with a View' begins with Lucy Honeychurch and her older cousin (and chaperone) Charlotte Bartlett arriving in Florence at their pensione, to the discovery that they were not given the rooms with a view, that they had been promised by the Signoria, but were given rooms far apart, looking onto a courtyard. They meet the socialist journalist Mr Emmerson and his son George, who has been brought up encouraged to be free-thinking uninfluenced by religions and superstition, that Forster comments lead men to hate each another in God's name. The father and son have rooms with views and insist they swap. Charlotte is initially against the room swap and insists Lucy does not have George's room as she knows where it would lead. For Lucy it leads to not only a room with a view but a relationship with George that entirely changes her own childhood room spatialisation, which is re-spatialised (*Stage 3*) into the new 'room' here. George represents freedom from all that had gone before including her childhood home. Just as Adela Quested searched for the 'real India', Lucy looked for the 'real Italy'. The real Italy was *Stage 1 – primal spatialisation*, pre- transferential, and, like the real India (and the Marbar Caves) can be experienced through primitive sensory experiences. The bohemian writer Miss Lavish described to Charlotte that she hopes to emancipate her from her Baedeker guide book and to go off the beaten path that is designated to find true adventure and the 'true Italy' and she also describes that every city has its own smell and that is an important part of the experience of Florence – the true Florentine smell. Forster gives a detailed description of Lucy's newly swapped room with a view, which is bright and bare, with a red-tiled floor and a painted ceiling.

It was also described how pleasing being able to open the windows is, to fling them far open and lean out and feel the sunshine and see the church, the trees, and the Arno flowing past. Lucy contrasts this experience with her home of Windy Corner where the road up through the woods to the house, the drawing room which is always clean and ordered and the view out over Sussex is pretty but seems like a pale replacement for this Italian experience. Forster likens this to the inability of a postcard to portray the reality of a real experience in a location.

It seems that the 'drawing room' at home represents the original site of her *Stage 2 Room-object*. This makes, not so much the Pensione in Florence 'drawing room', which is described by Forster as an attempt to replicate a Bloomsbury boardinghouse drawing room, (much like 'the Club' in Chandrapore relocates an interior that represents something unconnected to the actual country outside) and in this case does not represent the real Italy, but rather this replacement (bed) room with a view, seems to expend her psyche in a Stage 3 way, with an enlarged space of the view of Italy outside her bedroom representing the expansion and maturation.

Forster contrasts the real Italy with the church at Santa Croche, where Mr Emmerson remarks on the guide's comments that it was built by faith, saying that it was an opportunity not to pay workers appropriately. He also tends to a crying child who knocked against the marble effigy of a Bishop. Mt Emmerson likens this to the church generally. The effigy would be a *Stage 3* re-spatialised Room object, although in Chapter 8, p. 194 we will also be looking at effigies as Post Room-object spaces. Indeed, here Forster may be suggesting that the body of the church, itself is a Post Room-object space, like the colonial 'Club', the collective meaning of which is out-moded and dead, is a spatialised memory representing something that is gone, as set of spatialised ideas. This is contrasted with 'primal' elements when Lucy and George witness a man actually die in a fight in a Florentine square, a disturbing 'true Italy' scene. George then approaches her in the Florentine Loggia (a totally new kind of Primitive space of the real Italy) where he spontaneously kisses her.

Forster expresses the primal elements here referring to the idea that something of the spirit of the god Pan, not the original and great God Pan who he describes as being buried 2000 years, since Christianity took hold in the Community spatialising Psyche, but rather a little version of this god that has carried the spirit of mercurial wildness and spontaneity, that has primitive spatial aspects like that which exists in the Marbar Caves. In contrast to the church, this gets somehow re-introjected into the space but is closed down and Lucy retreats to the 'order' of Rome and Cecil Vyse, to whom she becomes engaged. Forster likens Cecil to a medieval gothic statue in contrast to the freedom and mischievousness of Pan. This takes place back in the 'drawing room' at home which is described by Forster as being the opposite of the Room with a view in Florence. Here in the Windy corner the heavy curtains, almost meeting the ground, are drawn to protect the new carpet from the sun, so the light filtering through was subdued. It is a room that feels restrained restricted, careful, and cossetted, in comparison with the Florence room, which feels wide open to the elements. Here, Lucy's original *Stage 2 Room-object* is retreated or regressed into and seems restrictive to progressing and living (the curtains are shut against glory of the sun and its primal power; it is 'tempered') unlike the room with a view, where the window is thrown open to the primal experience. Lucy eventually works out her 'muddle', realises that she loves George and chooses to live beyond the *Stage 2* room in the mature replacement *Stage 3* room with a view, on their honeymoon. Forster again uses Greek references, as with his description of Pan, in relation to the space of the Loggia. He refers to the room with a view in relation to the song of Phaerthon signifying that love has been attained between Lucy and George. However, at the end of the book, Forster also writes that Lucy and George were conscious of a mysterious and primitive love around the space of the room outside, relating to the river coming down from the melted winter snow in the mountains into the Mediterranean in the Spring; a primal spatial reference to the new beginning in the landscape around them.

Maurice; Early Queer Rooms and Spaces

Although in 'Maurice' Forster also makes comments on the church, what I shall be concentrating on here is, as David Leavitt wrote, 'E. M. Forster's Maurice is a novel without antecedents [...] it belongs to an age that knew almost nothing of what today we call, rather casually, 'gay fiction'' (Forster, 2012[1908], p. xi) – Forester's early queer room spaces, whilst dealing with 'classed' room spaces in relation to these. Maurice' childhood home was portrayed by Forster as being much like Windy Corner in 'A Room with a View' as he describes how Maurice's mother lived in a villa among some pines and that his father went to London to work every day. He described this as a 'land of facilities' (Forster, 2005[1971], p. 11), where no effort had to be made to get anything – the shops delivered and the station was nearby.

Forster gives a hint here of what Maurice considered un-striving – where there is plenty but perhaps not of the right things as he later considers that '[h]ome emasculated everything' (Forster, 2005[1971], p. 43). As with Windy Corner, this would be the original site of Maurice's original Primary spatialised Room-object activity (*Stage 2*), but for Maurice, his childhood bedroom is not all 'good' he describes his complex fear of seeing shadows in a mirror. Forster described Maurice's childhood bedroom as having a street lamp outside where the light shines through the curtains, sometimes in skull-like blots on the furniture. Maurice would find this terrifying even though all of the households were nearby. But at those times he would think about their servant George. The 'household' did not comfort him – perhaps they were part of the terror – the terror of emasculation and somehow a disappearance of his 'True self' (Winnicott, 1965, p. 140). Maurice's thinking about the servant George defends against this horror. Although George is the only other man in the house and this in itself would be a relief, it also hints at his relationship with Alec Scudder to come (Clive's 'servant') and with whom he finds 'home' at the end of the book. When Maurice visits the psychiatrist, Lasker Jones's consulting room, whilst under hypnotises, he has a *stage 3 Consulting Room-object* experience. This could have contained *stage 4* (including the transference to the therapist) elements. Maurice sees a picture on the consulting room wall that is initially suggested by the psychiatrist as being of a woman but Maurice formulates it into a man – the experience in the consulting room, seems in the end to affirm something new. We could see this as a *Stage 5* spatialisation where spatialisation in the consulting room is re-spatialised outside with Alec Scudder which, as with the room with a view in Florence for Lucy, seems to replace earlier experiences, and allows for maturation and growth of his psyche. Maurice's childhood 'inner landscape' is depicted as troubled as he is shown to be unable to have an understanding of his own sexuality that the society he grew up in would recognise. Forster utilises spatial landscape metaphors here again to describe Maurice's experience, of a darkness of night that was primeval yielding to dawn (the dawning realisation of his own sexuality) descending Valleys between smaller and larger mountains and pushing through fog. At Cambridge, Risley, who is more openly gay, seems to have a different inner landscape (Forster's metaphorical spatialised description are reminiscent of Freud's poetic landscape descriptions in Chapter 2, see p. 45) as, whilst Maurice was overshadowed by mountains in the valley, Risley was happily running around the summit of the mountain. He wondered if Risley would give him a hand up to the top of the mountain since he knew the route.

Maurice becomes clear about his sexuality through his relationship with Clive at Cambridge. When Clive whispered to Maurice that he loves him, Maurice was shocked to the bottom of 'his suburban soul'. (Forster, 2005[1971], p. 48) this shocks him out of the suburban home space and entering the room of Clive via the window, he enters a new space of possibilities and maturation. This is reflected in the landscape in a primal way. Forster again uses spatial landscape imagery to describe Maurice's experience with Clive, where they have a picnic in a landscape that is essentially fabricated and contrived by a human- there is a grassy embankment, water in a dyke above them, surrounded by landscaped willow trees. But at the same time although this landscape is created by humans, there is still something primitive and Stage 1 retained here – as Forster describes that 'man' who created the landscape is not there. Maurice and Clive can connect with the primal space of the landscape beyond that – like the Loggia in Italy or the Marbar cave – this transcends the human, contrived, and controlling value system and concepts, in this case a heterosexual, straight, imposing constriction is transcended.

However, the 'path' that Clive impressed upon them was a celibate one and though this was a narrow and beautiful path high above the metaphorical valley, it led to darkness again, not to the mountain summit. Clive abandons Maurice to take up his responsibilities in running his country estate Penge, managing game and tenants, with the objective of going into politics. Forster comments on this mismatch of society and reality, at Penge. Where all the men are smoking confidently after dinner as if they are in control of their estates and of the country and yet Maurice noticed that everything in the estate was in need of repair – the fences and gates, the window, and the floors. Here Forster is commenting on the ruling classes and whilst they arrange or rearrange (the people of) England, their own houses are in disrepair – a spatial metaphor for hypocrisy, in this case of gay men making themselves straight to order to fit with society or all people casting aside their own nature to conform to society, whilst their own natures are in 'disrepair' not attended to, ignores for the sake of the social needs. Forster also extends this to Colonialisation, as Clive's mother wants Clive to travel to the Colonies, which she sees as an essential part of society and business, indispensable in societising him as discussed earlier in relation to the colonial community (see p. 165). The state of the hypocritical room space continues, when Clive tells Maurice of his plans to get married to a woman, the words getting lost in the rain and making Maurice think about the dilapidated roofs at Penge that let in the rain. They are decayed and permeable like their relationship. Later at dinner, the roof metaphor comes in again when the drawing-room ceiling, 'dripped into basins and saucers' (Forster, 2005[1971], p. 153). This contrast with Maurice's mother's drawing room that is emasculating and Lucy Honeychurch's mother's drawing room that is oppressive and stifling, or the Florentine Pensione drawing room that is false and pretends to be something it is not. Here Clive's Penge, drawing room *(Stage 2)* is leaking everything, leaking integrity, and ruining all of its contents. Likewise Maurice's bedroom at Penge, the Russet Room threatens the same leaking, until Alec Scudder climbs through a window and opens up an entirely new *Stage 3* room space (or Stage 5 as discussed earlier). Alec was described as being of the woods, the water, and of fresh air – of the primal unrestricted wild landscape. Although Alec and Maurice meet up in the British Museum, amidst Colonial objects that belong to society, they are at home in the boating shed and take off into the wilderness to have a life together which Forster hoped would be a hopeful space in the future.

The Machine Stops; Forster's Virtual Room Spaces

Forster's 'The Machine Stops' is an uncannily predictive futuristic story that must, in 1928, have seemed impossibly far-fetched and out of this world, but, apart from many other science fiction novels and scripts being potentially influenced by it, many uncannily predictive aspects of life in the 2020s as well as features of the global Pandemic Covid-19, that my last Chapter 6 opens with; rooms, virtual rooms, communication, and the quality of mirroring afforded in these, are represented in the story. The story opens with the central character Vashti in her 'Room' which Forster describes as small and hexagonal like the cell in a beehive. It glows with soft light not from any obvious source, it has an air conditioning and heating system to keep it comfortable at all times like a womb, system. The only furniture is a desk and a chair in which sits the owner of the room, a woman called Vashti who is extremely white, due to her never having been outside. Her room gets Forster's characteristic graphic room deception and this gets added to throughout with more detail and spatial meanings as the story progresses. The room is one of millions under the surface of a post-apocalyptic earth where thousands of corridors covered in shiny tiles exist one tier upon another all containing millions of rooms.

In a later scene where Vashti is outside her room, she is afraid to be away from her comfort, security, and protection which her room (and 'the machine') provide contrasted because she believes that the cold of the air outside could kill her. For Vashti her room is shown to be everything that she cares for in the world, this room is Forster's version of what I am calling the *Stage 2 Room-object*. The Machine is the controlling mother of all, and the room and its walls are the manifestation of it. Children are raised in collective 'public' nurseries with occasion permitted visitations from their mothers, so Forster presents the nursery fulfilling of their needs being topped up by the 'room' as the 'The Room-object' space. The room perfectly mirrors the needs of the inhabitant, at the touch of a button – food, music, a bath with soapy bubbles, and a bed appears. In addition, the rooms are all exactly the same all over the world. When Vashti gets to her son's room, she discovers that it is exactly like her own in every way. That means there would be no *Stages 3–5* of my Room-object Spatial Matrix positions as there would be no need to re-spatialise – every room is the same Room-object space as if there is only one Room-object in the world; a manifestation spatially of the one mother machine. Punishment for wrongdoing is being made homelessness which effectively means death, as being outside in the wilderness and cold, which is fatally dangerous and cut off from the Room-object that provides all care and means of living. When Vashti considers leaving the room to visit her son, she pressed a button that she had not pressed before and the whole wall opened up. Vashti was terrified and ran back into the safely of her own room again.

So, leaving the room is worrying and Forster also played around with the significance of spatialising activity – and how this connects to ritual and belief. He shows that 'The Book of the Machine' (Forster, (2011[1928], p. 8), which she is comforted by, is an instructions manual for all that the machine provides, which, like a religious book, it is fashionable to richly bind. Vashti's son Kuno suggested that Vashti is starting to worship the machine. To which she replied that it is ridiculous as all the fear and superstition relating to religion have been removed by the machine. Forster is showing that spatialisation and ritualisation is innately human and that he has not been 'destroyed', but there is a re-establishment of religious belief and the people chant that the Machine is against superstition but that the Machine is eternal and all powerful. Forster, as I will discuss in Chapter 8, in relation to Freud and Balzac's magic skin see page 192), is saying something about too much projection meaning there is too much reliance on being inside the room and the Room-object. Forster says that space has been annihilated here and with it humans have lost part of themselves. Returning to the opening scene. Kuno rings his mother to ask her to visit him. We can already imagine that the mirroring between them was poor anyway (reflecting Forster own relationship with his mother- see Chapter 2, p. 40). We are told Vashti thinks about when he was taken away from her when he was a baby and put into a public nursery where she once visited him, he was then placed by the machine in a room on the other side of the world. But, given that their relationship and the mirroring for him with her is already greatly challenged, Forster then presents delightfully these virtual aspects of communication from the room that bizarrely predict the virtual aspect of working in Chapter 6. Kuno phones her to have a conversation and she is irritated as she is about to deliver a 'lecture' on Australian music on a social media platform. Forster's prediction in 1928 about having several thousand 'friends' that can be communicated with from their room like a social media type of communications, and where anyone can do five minutes lectures (like Vlogs) on anything to their audiences of social-media type followers, is extraordinary. Also, Forster's reference to 'isolate'; is uncanny. The word self-isolate became used in normal everyday language from 2020 during the pandemic. The mode of communication they used though, is most interesting. Forster predicted the form of communications from these rooms as being something like a video call on a tablet, laptop, or phone. Vashti holds a round plate that glows and the image of her son, who lives on the other side of the world, appears on it.

Forster then shows their challenged mirroring as Kuno asks his Mother to come and visit him in his room so he can speak to her about something important. She replies that she can see him, but he says that he wants to speak to her, not through the machine, and 'meet face to face and talk about the hopes that are in my mind'. (Forster, (2011[1928], pp. 3–4). Here there is a reference by Forster to meeting 'face to face' again, another phrase that since 2020 had been said constantly including within the virtual consulting room!

There is also a discussion by Kuno of his frustration of his Mother's lack of mirroring, as well the evaluation of the quality of the mirroring afforded by the machine screen. Interestingly, Vashti thought he looked sad but she could not be sure as 'the machine did not transmit *nuances* of expression' (Forster, (2011[1928], p. 5) but gave a general idea of people which Forster liken to the bloom on the grape being irreplicable in artificial grapes and that something 'good enough' had been accepted by humans that was not the real thing. This is reminiscent of his description in 'A Room with a View' that a postcard cannot adequately depict the experience of being in the space that the image is of.

This was not 'good enough' 'Mirroring' in a Winnicottian sense, though this was before Winnicott too! This mention of grapes is similar to Murphy's discussion of Sheryl Brahnam's, '"In-person communication resembles video conferencing about as much as a real blueberry muffin resembles a packaged blueberry muffin that contains not a single blueberry but artificial flavours" (Murphy, 2020), and is reminiscent of both Lemma's comment on the *'black mirror'* (Lemma, 2017, p. 47) that, 'technology is far from perfect: it introduced delays and distortions that undermine each party's confidence in what they can infer from what would otherwise be valuable cues such as the look on someone's face or the tone of their voice (Lemma, 2017, p. 91)' much like the experience of Kuno is communicating to Vashti. But Forster is very clear that there is a technology challenge to Mirroring but a more significant difficulty with Mirroring from his mother and the way in which she used the technology.

Conclusions

Forster presents many room spaces in his novels that have been analysed here through use of the Room-object Spatial Matrix to understand additional Psychosocial meanings that can be found in them. I am going to conclude this chapter, however, with a reflection on a thought Forster offers in 'The Machine Stops' when he discussed a future, social mediatised genericised virtualised approach to ideas, saying that 'first hand' ideas no longer exist as the general population are encouraged away from this to, if possible, 'tenth-hand' ideas which are safer and de-contaminated and removed from the dangerous and disturbing experience of real 'direct observation' (Forster, (2011[1928], p. 40). How wonderful that Forster encapsulated the essence of the difference between the safety in the Room-object and in known ideas with the 'disturbing element' of 'direct observation' that we have observed in the *Stage 1* moments for patients when a direct experience manifests a *Stage 1* spatialiased sensory memory of real experience. Freud discusses these sorts of locational direct experiences in Paris and Forster in Florence and India. Here in this book, I tentatively attempt to get close in to this direct observation and direct ideas that are an essential element of both the Physical and the Virtual consulting room and what stops it being like the 'artificial' grapes.

Figure References

Figure 7.1: The Ruined Mosque. Drawing by D. Wright.

Figure 7.2: The Marbar Caves. Painting by D. Wright.

Figure 7.3: Howards End. Drawing by D. Wright.

References

Brahnam S. (2017) Comparison of In-Person and Screen-Based Analysis Using Communication Models: A First Step Toward the Psychoanalysis of Telecommunications and Its Noise, *Psychoanalytic Perspectives*. 14, Issue 2 Technology.

Cesaire, A. (2000) Discourse on Colonialism, Translated by Joan Pinkhamin *A Poetics of Anti Colonialism* by Robin D. G.. Kelley, N.Y: Monthly Review Press.

Davids F. (2002) September 11th 2001: Some Thoughts on Racism and Religious Prejudice as an obstacle, *British Journal of Psychotherapy*. 18(3):361–366.

Eliade, M. (1959) The Sacred and the Profane the Nature of Religion. (Trans. Trask, W.R.). New York and London: Harcourt Brace & Jovanovich.

Fanon F. (1963 [1961]) *The Wretched of the Earth* NY Grove Weidenfeld: Grove Press.

Forster E. M. (2012 [1908]) *A Room with a View*, London: Penguin.

Forster, E. M. (2012 [1910]) *Howards End*, London: Penguin.

Forster, E. M. (1985 [1924]) *A Passage to India*, London: Penguin.

Forster E. M. (2005 [1971]) *Maurice*, London: Penguin.

Forster, E. M. (2011 [1928]) *The Machine Stops*. London: Penguin.

Gilbert H. & Tompkins, J. (1996) *Post-Colonial Drama: Theory, Practice, Politics*, London, Routledge.

Kandiyoti D. (2002) Post-Colonialism Compared: Potentials and Limitations in the Middle East and Central Asia, *International Journal of Middle East Studies*. 34, 279–297. Printed in the United States of America.

Klein, M. (1946) Notes on Some Schizoid Mechanisms. The International Journal of Psycho-Analysis, 27: 99–110.

Kohon, G. (1999) *The Dead Mother*, London & NY: Routledge.

Lemma, A. (2017) *The Digital Age on the Couch Psychoanalytic practice and New Media*. London & New York: Routledge.

Massey, D. (2005) *For Space* London: Sage.

Moore-Gilbert, B. (1997) *Postcolonial Theory: Contexts, Practices and Politics*, London: Verso.

Murphy, K. (2020) Why Zoom Is Terrible There's a reason video apps make you feel awkward and unfulfilled. *The New York Times Sunday Review* https://www.nytimes.com/2020/04/29/Sunday-review/zoom-video-conference.html

Sartre, J. (1963) Preface to Fanon F. (1963 [1961]) *The Wretched of the Earth* (NY Grove Weidenfeld: Grove Press).

Winnicott, D. W. (1965) The Maturational Processes and the Facilitating Environment: Studies in the Theory of Emotional Development, *The International Psycho-Analytical Library*, 64: 1–276. London: The Hogarth Press and the Institute of Psycho-Analysis.

Wollheim, R. (1969) "The Mind and the Mind's Image of Itself". *International Journal of Psycho-Analysis*. 50: 209–220.

Wright, D. (2018) Rooms as Replacements for People: The Consulting Room as a Room Object (pp. 251–262). In: *On Replacement – Cultural, Social and Psychological Representations*. Editors: Owen, J. and Segal, N., Switzerland: Palgrave Macmillan.

Wright, D. (2019) Spatialisation and the Fomenting of Political Violence (pp. 167–187). In: *Fomenting Political Violence – Fantasy, Language, Media, Action*. Editors: Kruger, S., Figlio, K. and Richards, B., Switzerland: Palgrave Macmillan.

Chapter 8

The End Chapter, the End Room-object and Post Room-object Spaces; Conclusions of Clinical and Psychosocial Considerations of the Room-object Spatial Matrix

This chapter will reflect on the book as a whole, as well as the End Room-object, which I suggest as an additional stage to the Room-object Spatial Matrix, where the de-formation and de-spatialising of objects process, that is the opposite of the spatialised object formation at the beginning of life, will be looked at. I also look at the Post Room-object space. As with the de-spatialising of the object formation at the end, this chapter goes back through the stage of the book to the theoretical element of construction of the Room-object space, in Chapters 3, 2, then 1.

The Room-object Spatial Matrix Stage 6 – End Room-object Space

I will now discuss here my introduction of the sixth position on the Room-object Spatial Matrix. I suggest that at the end, object relating can go back to the beginning; life begins with the spatialising of parts of mother to function and at the end there is a de-spatialising and a letting go of the need to spatialise – the relinquishing and de-formation of objects. I suggest that this can also happen with the Room-object space – the de-spatialisation and de-construction of Room-objects can lead to *End Room-object* spaces. I have argued that a part of the formation of objects is spatialisation. Here, in this final room, the objects can be de-constructed/de-formulated, and the objects and Room-objects are likewise de-spatialised, as if returning to being unborn or unliving.

I have been particularly contemplating this conceptualisation since the experience of observing my mother's end-room process. I made a series of drawings, similar in process to the drawings that I made in my exploration, countertransferentially, of the Room-object Spatial Matrix in Chapter 3 (shown in Figs. 3.1–3.5), one of which I will use here to illustrate this end stage, along with a lino-cut print showing the pre-ending, de-spatialisation process. This End Room-objects space could be thought of as being an additional sixth stage on the Room-object Spatial Matrix- *Stage 6- End-Room object.*

DOI: 10.4324/9781003188117-8

In the case of my mother, in the last few weeks when the cancer that she had in her lungs and liver had spread up to her brain, she was cared for in a small NHS hospital. The first period of this time involved regressive elements to being very in touch with the Room-object Matrix *Stage 1 – Primitive spatialising* where the room space dominates in either a 'good' or 'bad' *Room-object* way. I am suggesting that the projection onto and spatialisation of room spaces that can oscillate between good and bad, as can be seen in Chapters 4, 5, and 6, particularly manifests when the pressure of (consulting) room moves generate unexpected *Stage 1 Primal Spatialisation* elements, creating a splitting of good and bad rooms stimulated by intense sensory experiences.

Good and Bad Room-object Spaces

We can think of these intense sensory experiences as regressive and spatialising as a defensive and protective functioning, which I suggest all humans do under pressure, and in particular we have observed this in relation to Room-object spaces and moves. In this case of the ending room with my mother, Fig. 8.1 depicts an ambivalent and oscillating Room-object space where there is an oscillation between a perception of the Room-object space being bad (and anxious, threatening, unsafe) and my mother being distressed by it, trying to get away from it and intensely disliking it, and to good Room-object space that feels containing and caring (comforting and embracing, almost disappearing into the bedclothes) see Fig. 8.2. In relation to the Bad Room-object space – this is very understandable – having to be away from home and in a strange room, that process feeling out of control and imposed, would as seen in Chapters 4, 5, and 6, create a 'Bad' room–move experience. In addition, though, as a young child, in the 1940s, my mother had spent a year in hospital after being run over by a car whilst playing on a tricycle. She endured a shattered pelvis and was in traction for a year, whilst also, at times, being isolated due to scarlet fever and chickenpox outbreaks. Her experience of being in hospital rooms must have, at times, been very frightening, lonely, and isolating. However, at other times in this ending stage, the room seemed to be a good Room-object for my mother, the space seemed to be embracing – like the Henri Rey's 'brick mother' (Steiner [in Rey], 1994, p. ix) (see p. 78) containing hospital setting.

After my mum passed away, I found a folder of very poignant letters that my mother had written to her mother from hospital in the 1940s as a young child. She had managed to make the hospital a good 'brick mother' and told her mother of the soft toys that she was making with the nurses and she had drawn pictures of the hospital and her house, telling her mother not to worry and that she was fine. This shows an early ability to make things and spaces good and split of the bad for her mother, in presenting the good in her letters.

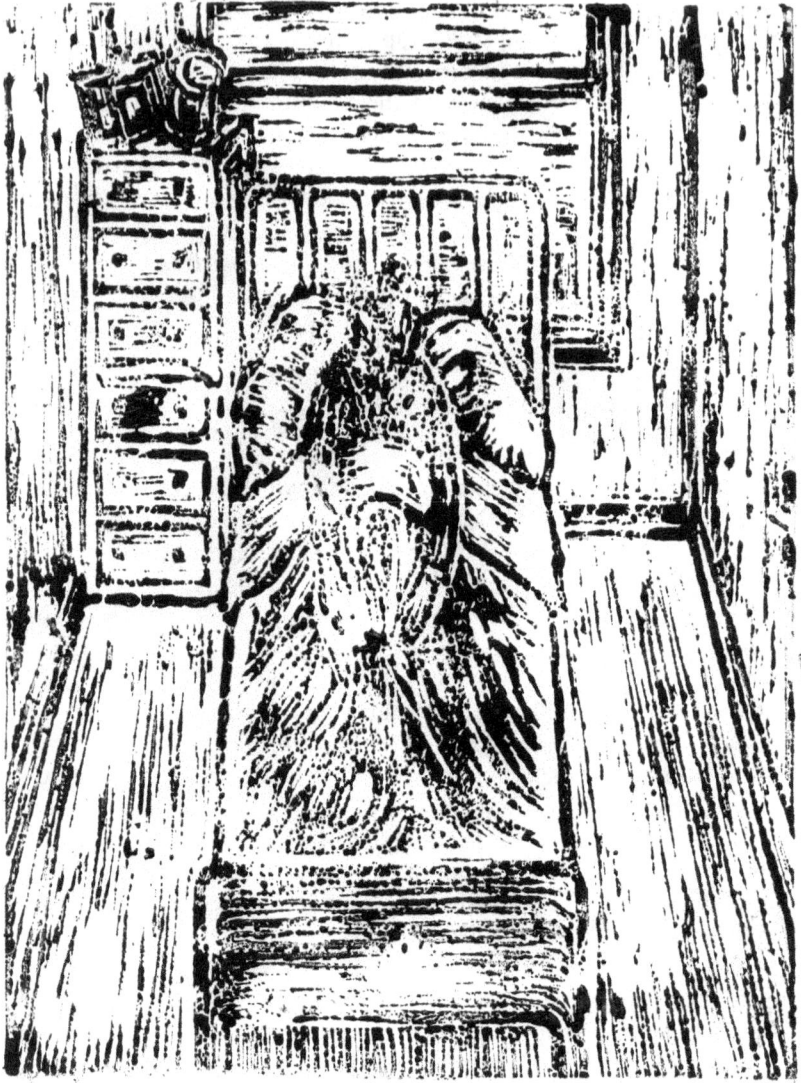

Figure 8.1 In the ending room – the re-spatialised early bad room space, (Stage 1 of the Room-object Spatial Matrix– Primal Spatialising). Lino cut print by D. Wright.

The End Room-object

After the phase of good and bad Room-object oscillation, the next phase that could be seen was the *End Room-object*. My drawing in Fig. 8.2 depicts this, where my mother seemed to de-object-relate, de-spatialise,

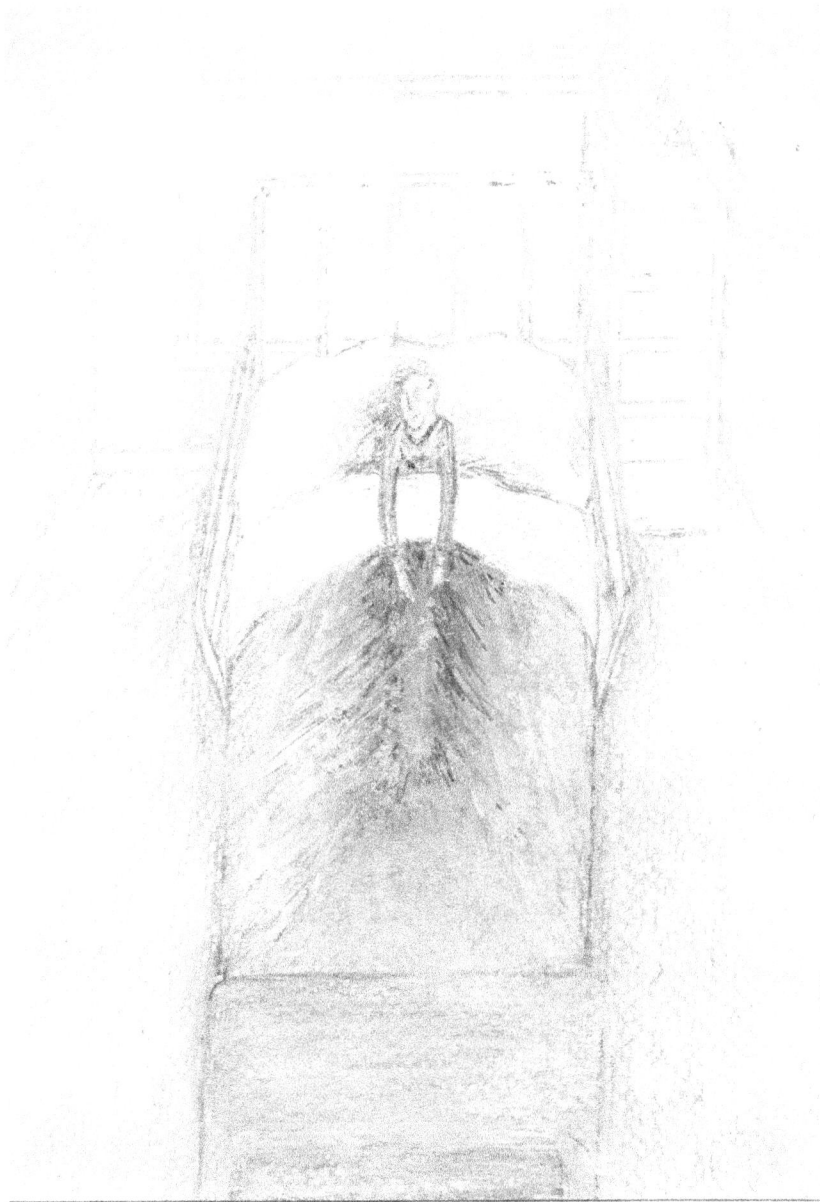

Figure 8.2 The End Room-object. Drawing by D. Wright.

de-Room-object spatialise. The room was neither good or bad, it did not matter anymore, there was an internalisation, much like maternal pre-occupation during pregnancy or with a baby, in this case with the self. We could say that it is a self-maternal pre-occupation that replaces and does away with the need for the internal and spatialised objects. These objects, parts of mother spatialised to create these internal objects, are no longer necessary for functioning and with them the Room-object space is no longer as important and spatialiased in the same way – it does not matter anymore.

Clinical Example of the End Room-object: Mr A

Returning to Mr A from Chapter 1 (see page 20), Mr A described the end process of his partners' mother at the end of her struggle with Cancer. She was back home from the hospital in the last 2 weeks, and spent most of her time sitting in her sitting room, on a special chair provided by the hospital to support her. Here she received family and friends who visited to see her. Mr A described how she became gradually less engaged in the process of engaging with the visitors of the space. Where once she would have been very engaged in the making of her space being good for visitors, as well as making food and hosting, she could not do that. Instead Mr A facilitated this process of visitors and making the sitting room nice for them as well as providing refreshments for the visitors to support both his partner and partner's mother. We could think of this as the Winnicottian father's role whilst the mother experiences maternal preoccupation, the father looks after the environment for the mother and the baby. Here Mr A facilitated the process of looking after the environment (*End Room-object* space) for his partner who became the carer and his partner's mother – who was enabled to have this pre-occupation process that I described above as part of the de-object and de-spatialising experience of the Stage 6 – *End-Room object* space. Over the 2 weeks, Mr A reported this feeling of his partners' mother withdrawing from caring anymore about the room space and the items in it, as this *End room-object* experience took place.

Andre Gide's Mother in the End Room-object Space

Andre Gide's account of his Mother's *End Room-object* Space, in his autobiographical work, 'If It die' (using Dorothy Bussy's translation of 1957) provides a comprehensive example of the processes involved, where at the end, for his mother, there is a process of relinquishing control of rooms and space that had been so important to her and we could say a gradual lessening of the spatialisation processes visibly, of spaces and things in them. In chapters prior to his Mother's *End Room-object* space, Gide describes in intricate detail, the importance of the rooms of his family home and his mother's control of them, particularly her drawing room, where she had complete control over the space and put an enormous amount of effort into furnishing (which is described by Gide in great detail) as well as preparing for visitors, which he depicts as meaningful and we might think of as spatialising. Gide, like Sigmund Freud, (in Chapter 2) is very interested in maternal and paternal aspects of space (the paternal being Gide's father's library and study); however, for the purposes of thinking here about his mother's End-Room-object space, I will concentrate on Gide's detailed description of his mothers' spatialising investment in the space of her drawing room, and how this can be seen to contrast with her End Room-object experience. Gide writes that it was not a room that he went into often as it was her space and contained her things ordered in the way that she liked: 'The room was usually kept half shut up; and the furniture carefully protected by loose covers of white dimity, finely stripped with bright red. These covers so exactly fitted the chairs and sofas, that it was a pleasure putting them on again every Thursday morning after Wednesday's ceremonial – for Wednesday was my mother's 'at home' day' (Gide [Trans. Dorothy Bussy], 1987, p. 134). Gide described in great detail the items that his mother had in her drawing room such as the candelabra, clock, and chandeliers, 'imitation Louis XVI armchairs, upholstered in blue and gold damask', grand chairs by the fireplace 'whose grandeur was absolutely dazzling' with gilt on black, which he described that he was not allowed to sit on. He then describes the silk floral cross-stick fireplace screen which had particular spatialised meaning for his mother who 'had worked it secretly in the early days of her married life; entering the study on his birthday one morning, my father had been met by the startling sight. Gentle as he was and adoring my mother, he had almost lost his temper: 'No, Juliette,' he had cried; 'no, I beg of you. This is my study. Let me arrange this room at any rate in my own way.' Then, recovering his good-humour, he had persuaded my mother that although he liked the screen very much, he preferred seeing it in the drawing-room. (Gide [Trans. Dorothy Bussy], 1987, pp. 135–136).

This gives us a detailed picture of his mother's relationship with the space of her 'drawing-room', the house, and how skilled, tasteful, and vigorous she was in her eye for detail and design. We can say she was spatialising in the space as well in décor as the effort to prepare the rooms for visits and his not being allowed on the chair. This sets the scene for his description of her *End Room-object space* and the relinquishing of this spatialising, of her continual striving, creating what he described she 'thought lovely or worthy to be loved' whatever her object drives that led her to do that. He wrote that his mother had a stroke and was lying in a bed in the big room that she preferred. He found her there and he described this End Room-object scene in great detail;

> I am almost sure she recognised me; but she did not have clear idea of the time or the place or of herself or of the people around her; for she

showed neither surprise nor pleasure at seeing me. Her face was not much changed, but her eyes were vague and her features so expressionless that it seemed although her body no longer belonged to her and she has ceased to control it. It was so strange that I felt more amazement than pity. She was in a half-sitting position, propped up by pillows; her arms were outside the bed clothes and she was trying to write in a large open account-book. Even now her restless desire to intervene, to advise, to persuade, was still troubling her; she seemed in great mental agitation, and the pencil she held in her hand ran over the blank sheet of paper, but without making any mark; and the uselessness of this supreme effort was inexpressively distressing. I tried to speak to her, but my voice did not reach her; and when she tried to speak herself, it was impossible for me to make out what she wanted to say. I took away the paper in the hope she might be able to rest, but her hand continued to write on the sheets. At last she drowsed off and her features gradually relaxed; her hands ceased moving.

(Gide [Trans Dorothy Bussy] 1987, pp. 302–303)

Here, in this *Stage 6 End- room space*, in the room 'she preferred' she no longer had a clear idea of the time, place, or those around her and there is a kind of fading out of her spatialising activity in the bed she as the de-objects processes that I suggest relate to a de-Room-object process of letting go of 'control' and spatialising. The detail in which Gide described his observations is both touching and also allows this process that I am calling the *End room-object* to be shown. Naomi Segal examines Gide's rich and complex imagery in his writing (Segal 1998) and Jacques Lacan discussed the very detailed way in which Gide writes 'the room he makes for the comedy that structures things: Assuming that the tone he adopts in it surprises the reader in remaining devoid of affectation while running parallel to the modulation, which is one-of-a-kind, [...] of what in Gidian terms I would call the most tender attention. For this is clearly the kind of attention that leads him to revive somewhere the archaic genitive of the "Gide childhoods."' (Lacan (2002[1966], p. 625). Gide's description of his mother's End Room-object space that he has observed shown in stark contrast by Gide's detailed rendering of her care and spatialising control of her drawing-room was extremely poignant and evocative. Lacan also writes about the relationship 'between Gide and his mother' who Lacan describes as a 'maternal figure wrought by psychologizing pedantry'. (Lacan Fink and Grigg (2002[1966], p. 629) As pedantry is an excessive concern with minor details and rules, we can say that this not only relates to what Lacan calls her 'moral mothering' ((Lacan Fink and Grigg (2002[1966], p. 625) but it relates to the detail that she put into her own spatialising construction – that Gide had understood and was a witness to in her life and at the end. At the end, Gide reflects on this control that his mother exerted in the space, with a new perspective in which he, '[a]dmired her for her life which had been one continual effort to draw a little nearer to what she thought lovely or worthy to be loved. I was alone in the big room, alone with her, watching the solemn approach of death, and feeling the restless beatings of that unflagging part re-echo in my own. (Gide [Trans Dorothy Bussy], 1987, p. 304). In the front of his book, it reads, 'Except a corn of wheat fall into the ground and die, it abideth alone: But if it die, it bringeth forth much fruit. John 12, 24. This may be about the End time of his mother and the fruit brought forth by his reflections and understanding of her at and after the end, and therefore perspective on living the rest of his life which may perhaps have been experienced by him as liberating in relation to his own object relating. This relates to further to- wards the end of this chapter, where I discuss *Post Room-object* spaces, which I suggest is off the end of the Room-object matrix stages, it is after death and after object relating, relating to either individual projected post- death object spatialising and/or connected to others post-death spatialising of the person. Gide's account in his book 'If It die' is a Post-object account.

Returning to E.M. Forster from the previous chapter, where we ended with the bad mirroring from the mother in the Virtual room in 'The Machine Stops'. David Leavitt discussed Gide as well as Balzac, who I will be discussing in the next section. Leavitt suggests that Foster's sexuality and ability to live the life he wanted was restricted by his Mother in a way Gide's was not because she had already died;

> E. M. Foster's Maurice is a novel without antecedents [...] it belongs to an age that knew almost nothing of what today we call, rather casually, 'gay fiction' [...] When he sat down to write Maurice, Foster had probably read Andre Gide's The Immortalist (1902) as well as Balzac's Lost Illusions [...]. In his life as well as in his art, he was an ambivalent revolutionary, enmeshed in a network of social and sexual rigidities which he criticised but made no real effort to transcend. Thus he rose to the defence of Radclyffe Hall's lesbian novel The Well of Loneliness, and cultivated a circle the members of which included numerous male couples; but he also carried over from his family- which was more middle class than he would have liked- to tendency to conventionality. His mother, he wrote in his diary, was 'deeply shocked' by Howards End [...]. Later, when his friend J.R. Ackerley urged him to be more open about his homosexuality, by pointing out the contrary example of Gide, he replied, 'But Gide hasn't got a mother!'
>
> (Leavitt D, in Forster 2012[1908]: pp. xi–xiv)

Forster's mother character, Vashti, who in 'The Machine Stops', shows bad mirroring and intense controlling of the room spaces and of her sons thinking and behaviours in relation to 'The machine', may relate to his re- lationship with his own mother and as well as Forster's potential to be empathic with room spaces, that are portrayed in such graphic and wonderful detail in his novels. Leavitt's reference to Balzac, now leads us on to the next section in relation to Sigmund Freud's End Room-object space and his last novel he read in it; Balzac's La Peau de chagrin.

Sigmund Freud and the End Room-object Space Process in the Consulting Room

We will now return to Sigmund Freud's relationship with rooms, following on from Chapter 2, in this, his last room, his *End Room-object* space, that he would spend his last weeks in and passed way in; his consulting room in Maresfield Road. After the de-construction of Freud's consulting room in Berggasse (as depicted in Engelman's photographs, see Figures 2.10, 2.11 and 2.13) Freud came to London and began his last life chapter. Jones writes of Freud's feelings of triumph and belonging in relation to his arrival in London,

> I drove past Buckingham palace and Burling ton House to Piccadilly Circus and up Regent Street, Freud eagerly identifying each landmark and pointing it out to his wife. [...]. During the night journey from Paris to London he dreamt that the was landing at Pevensey [...] where William the Conqueror had landed in 1066. This did not sound like a depressed refugee, and indeed it foreshadowed the almost royal honours with which he was greeted in England.
>
> (Jones, 1967[1953], pp. 647–648)

We see here, the spatialisation that Jones portrays Freud to have much like his spatialising to the meaning of Paris and Notre dame in relation to Charcot (see Page 44) and also his utilising of feeling about Monuments in London to describe Mnemic symbols (Freud, (1957 [1910]). (see p. 31) which I will also discuss again further on in this chapter, in his formulation of London as a place to make a home in. Jones goes on to write of Freud's experience in his new consulting room and his new home at Maresfield Gardens (his consulting room shown in my drawing in Fig. 8.3, through the right hand windows):

> he was highly pleased with it. He said it was too good for someone who would not tenant it for long, but it was really beautiful [...]. His consulting-room, filled with his loved possessions, opened through French windows directly on to the garden – the very spot where a year later he died. His son Earnst had arranged all pictures and the cabinets of antiquities to the best possible advantage in a more spacious way than had been feasible in Vienna, and Paula's memory enabled her to replace the various objects on Freud's desk in their precise order, so that he felt at home the moment he sat at it on his arrival. All his furniture, books, and

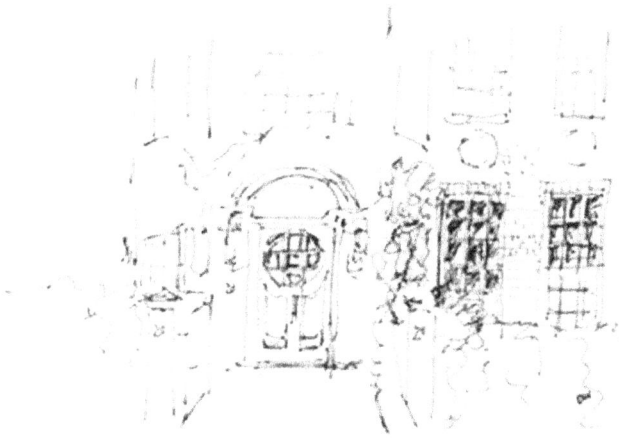

Figure 8.3 Sigmund Freud's Consulting Room from the front- 20 Maresfield Gardens, Drawing by D. Wright.

antiquities had arrived safely in London on 15 August, and in his large consulting room, or study, everything was excellently arranged to display his beloved possessions to their best advantage.'

(Jones, 1967[1953], pp. 647–648)

This re-spatialised *Room-object space/Consulting room-object space*, was re-created, re-spatialiased for his arrival, with care from everyone to make it good and like Berggasse. Perhaps too because although this space was to be a re-spatialised version of the Room-object space (and original psychoanalytic Consulting room-object space of all consulting rooms) we considered (see page 41) that this Room-object space was a spatialised Room-objects space of the 'cabinet' – his childhood bedroom, and it was also soon to be his *End Room-object* space.

The End Room-object Space, Final Objects, and the Mahogany Couch

As Jones wrote, 'His consulting-room, filled with his loved possessions, opened through French windows directly on to the garden – the very spot where a year later he died' (Jones, 1967, pp. 647–648). Jones went on to describe the end:

'We approach the end. The anxious feature now was that in the last 2 years suspicious areas no longer proved to be pre-cancerous leucoplakias, but definitely malignant recurrences of the cancer itself.

At Christmas 1938 Schur removed a sequestrum of bone, the one about whose existence Freud had become doubtful, and this gave considerable relief. But at the same time a swelling appeared and gradually took on an increasingly ominous look. Professor Lacassagne, the Director of the Curie Institute in Paris, was fetched and made an examination on 26 February. He could not advocate radium treatment, however. A Biopsy had disclosed an unmistakable malignant recurrence, but the surgeons decided it was inaccessible and that no further operation was feasible [...] The end was in sight. Only palliative treatment remained [...] In August everything went downhill rapidly. He was getting very week and spent his time in a sick bay in his study from which he could gaze at the flowers in the garden.

(Jones, 1967[1953], pp. 651–656)

So here in his Study/Consulting room, his End room-object space- he spent his final days at the windows at the back, on the mahogany couch/ bed shown here in the photograph in Fig. 8.4, provided by the Freud Museum. On the occasions that this final couch has been in display in the Freud Museum the interpretation stated; *The Couch upon which Sigmund Freud Died. In the final weeks of Freud's life, this mahogany couch was moved into his study. Too ill to climb the stairs, he lay in this*

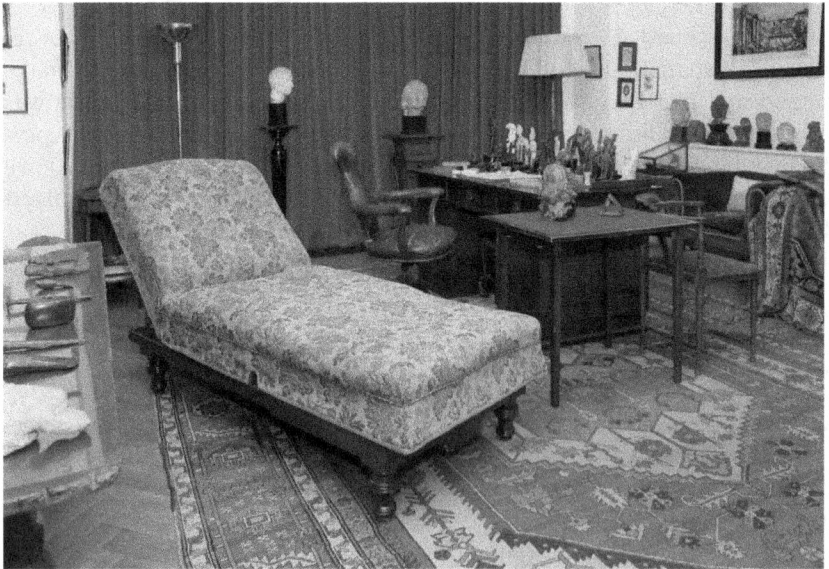

Figure 8.4 The Couch upon which Sigmund Freud spent his final days and on which he died. Photograph © Freud Museum London.

room surrounded by his family, his doctors and, of course, his antiquities. Eventually, in the early morning of 23rd September 1939, the 83-year-old Sigmund Freud, assisted by an injection of morphine, died on his invalid couch, only a few feet away from the most famous carpeted and cushioned psychoanalytical couch.

Balzac's La Peau de chagrin – Last Book Freud Read; Skin on the Walls and Room-object at the End

Jones wrote of Freud's last book that he read in this End Room-object space; 'The last book he was able to read was Balzac's La Peau de chagrin, on which he commented wryly: 'That is just the book for me. It deals with starvation.' He meant rather the gradual shrinking, the becoming less and less, described so poignantly in the book.' (Jones, 1967[1953], p. 656). Honoré de Balzac novel of 1831, 'La Peau de chagrin', which in the English translation is called, The Wild Ass's Skin, is set in early-nineteenth century Paris. It is the story of a young man who, after hitting difficult times financially and losing his last gold coin in a gambling house, decides to kill himself in the Seine after nightfall. Whilst waiting for night to fall he walks done towards it, on the way, a scene that, like the Gambling house Balzac describes in great detail;

> He walked with melancholy step alongside the shops, listlessly examining the merchandise displayed. When the shops came to an end he studied the Louvre, the Institute, the towers of Notre-Dame, the turrets of the Palace and the Pont des Arts. These monuments appeared to be taking on a dreary look as they reflected the grey tints of the sky, whose rare gleams of sunlight imparted a menacing air to Paris.
>
> (Balzac, 1977[1831], p. 32)

This scene is reminiscent of Freud's own description of the 'monuments' of London (Freud, (1957[1910]) as Mnemic symbols, (see p. 31) as I have just discussed and will also discuss below. Here, Balzac not only has the monuments representing a spatial array of spatialised emotions for the central character, here, in Paris, which, as discussed in Chapter 2, Paris was also a very important location for Freud as was Notre Dame mentioned here by Balzac. Balzac then goes on to give a detailed account of the interior and contents of the 'old curiosity shop' that the young man comes across comes, 'to pass the time before nightfall [...] At first sight, the show-rooms offered him a chaotic medley of human and divine works. Crocodiles, apes, and stuffed boas grinned at stained glass windows.' (Balzac, 1977[1831], pp. 33–34).

The shopkeeper tells the young man:

> Without offering you anything whatsoever in gold, silver, bullion, bank
> notes or letters of credit, I propose to make you richer, more powerful
> and more respected than a king can be [...] 'Turn round,' said the dealer,
> suddenly seizing the lamp in order to direct its light onto the wall
> opposite the picture. 'Look at that WILD ASS'S SKIN,' he added. The
> young man stood up abruptly and showed some surprise as he espied
> above the seat on which he was sitting a piece of shagreen fastened to
> the wall, not exceeding the dimensions of a fox's pelt. But, thanks to a
> phenomenon which at first he could not explain, this skin projected,
> from amid the deep darkness which reined in the shop such luminous
> rays that you might have thought they emanated from a small comet.
>
> (Balzac, 1977[1831], pp. 49–50).

This magic untanned skin from a wild ass (shagreen) promises to fulfil his
every desire, but each time it grants a wish (particularly relating to power),
the skin shrinks and with it the physical energy of the owner. The Young
man does not take the shop keepers advice and ends rich, but exhausted and
decrepit.

The story is striking in many ways in relation to the theses of this
chapter – not least in the skin on the wall in the scene of the shop. The
engraving in Fig. 8.5 from the title page of the first edition of the book
shows this well as the magic skin, across the wall, glows in luminosity. This
takes us back to Chapter 3 and the original formulation of the Room-
object Spatial Matrix, during which; Bick [Skin], Anziou [Skin-ego], and
Rey [Brick mother] were considered) and in the Stage 2 Room-object space
illustration (Figure 3.2, page 80) the wallpaper is shown as mother's skin.
Thus, related to for example Ms B's experience is discussed (see page 74 &
98) of early object formation, part- object-mother's skin, and Mr E's
concerns about the plastering of the walls in the renovates house; a created
Stage 5 Room-object space/mother.

According to Jones, Freud reads the book and he laughs about
'shrinking'. Freud's cancer was diminishing him and 'shrinking' him – as
well as perhaps a de-constructing and de-spatialised in this End Room-
object space. The text on Balzac's magic skin reads 'Possess me and thou
shalt possess all things but thy life is forfeit to me (Balzac, 1977[1831],
pp. 49–51)'. Freud is perhaps giving a hint to thinking about this *End room-
object* space, that a life lived through projection and transference, though
part of the original object (and Room-object) functioning for survival (it
saves the protagonist in the book from death) when it is without consciousness, as Klein warns about, excessive schizoid projection – there is a
depletion of the self.

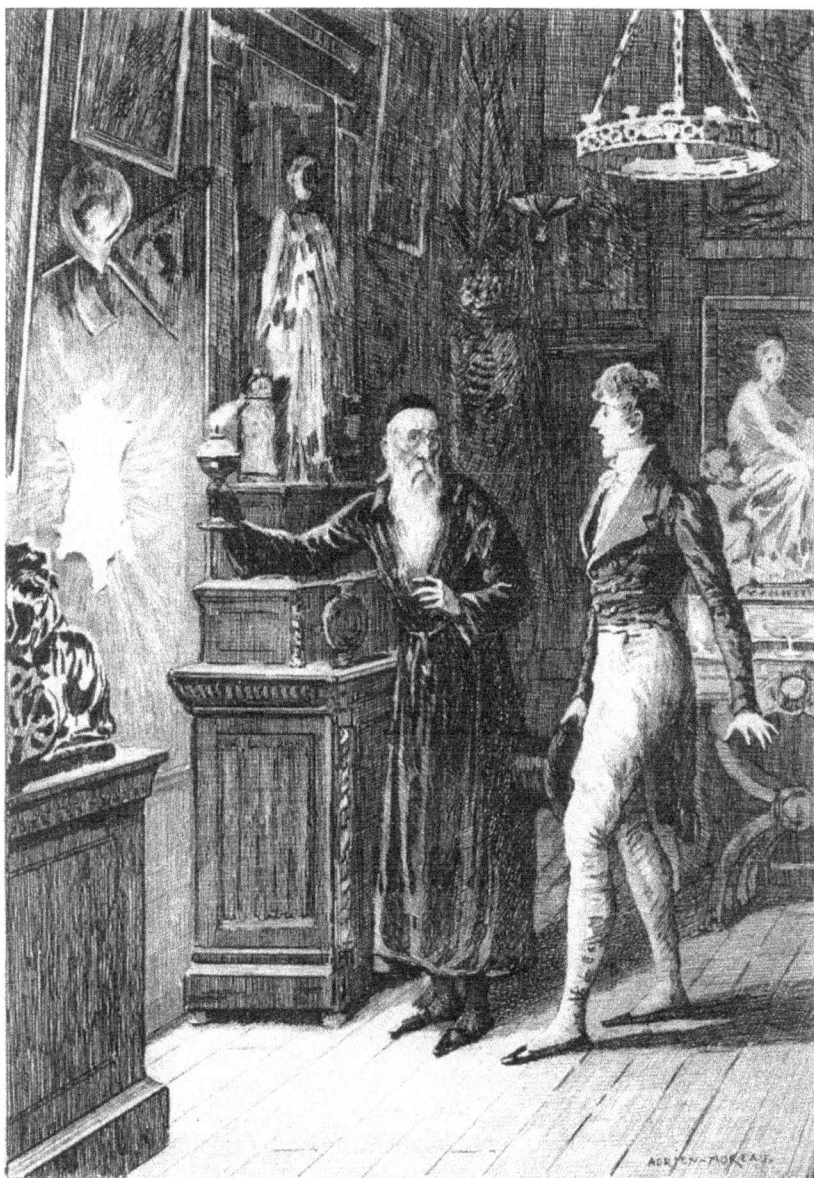

Figure 8.5 Engraving by Adrien Moreau from the title page of Honoré de Balzac's The Magic Skin (1897).

After the Room-object Spatial Matrix; The Post-life, Post Room-object Space

This leads on to what I am calling the Post Room-object space, shown here in my lino-cut print, Fig. 8.6 showing a post-death room with my Mother. We can think of this as being beyond the Room-object Spatial Matrix, it is what comes after, which could be a planned projected meaning of the self, combined with an individual or collective post-death spatialising relating to them. This links back to Chapter 1 and the space of the Rising Star Cave – with early hominin 'body disposal' suggesting ritual and spatialiased meaning as well as spaces in Westminster Abbey. I have written (Wright 2018) on Ernst Kantorowicz's thinking on this post-end, and what I am thinking here as *Post Room-object* space:

> Ernst Kantorowicz writes of the case of kings, who have many fantasies projected onto them by members of society relating to their position as protector of the cohesion of that society. When he dies his physical body dies and the projected meanings pass onto a replacement physical body – the King is dead, long live the King. There is then an issue of what to do with the physical body as it contradicts the symbolism of the immortal body. Society had to create 'new fictions' (314) to protect against this potential threat to cohesion. One of these fictions involved covering up the dead body with a monument in the form of an image of the body, often in the walls of a chapel in a cathedral or abbey. Here again the walls are marked out with replacement imagery to maintain control.
>
> (Wright, 2018, p. 253)

Kantorowicz discussed the function of tombs as a spatialisation for the viewer, not the deceased, although they may have a projected aspiration of spatialisation whilst still alive. In the case of the medieval royals and dignitaries who had these tombs spaces made into the walls of Westminster Abbey and became part of the space of the building inside, as well as having an enduring representations of themselves which in the case of the king or queen fulfils the function of continuity between dead/alive, as Kantorowicz discusses, 'The King never dies' and 'By interpreting the People as an universitas "which never dies" the jurisprudents had arrived at the concept of a perpetuity of both the whole body politic (head and members together) and the constituent members alone.' (Kantorowicz, 1997[1957], p. 314).

The Post Room-object Space of Eleanor of Castille

An example of this from Westminster Abbey would be the tomb of Eleanor of Castille (see Fig. 8.7), who lived 1241 to 1290. At her death, her

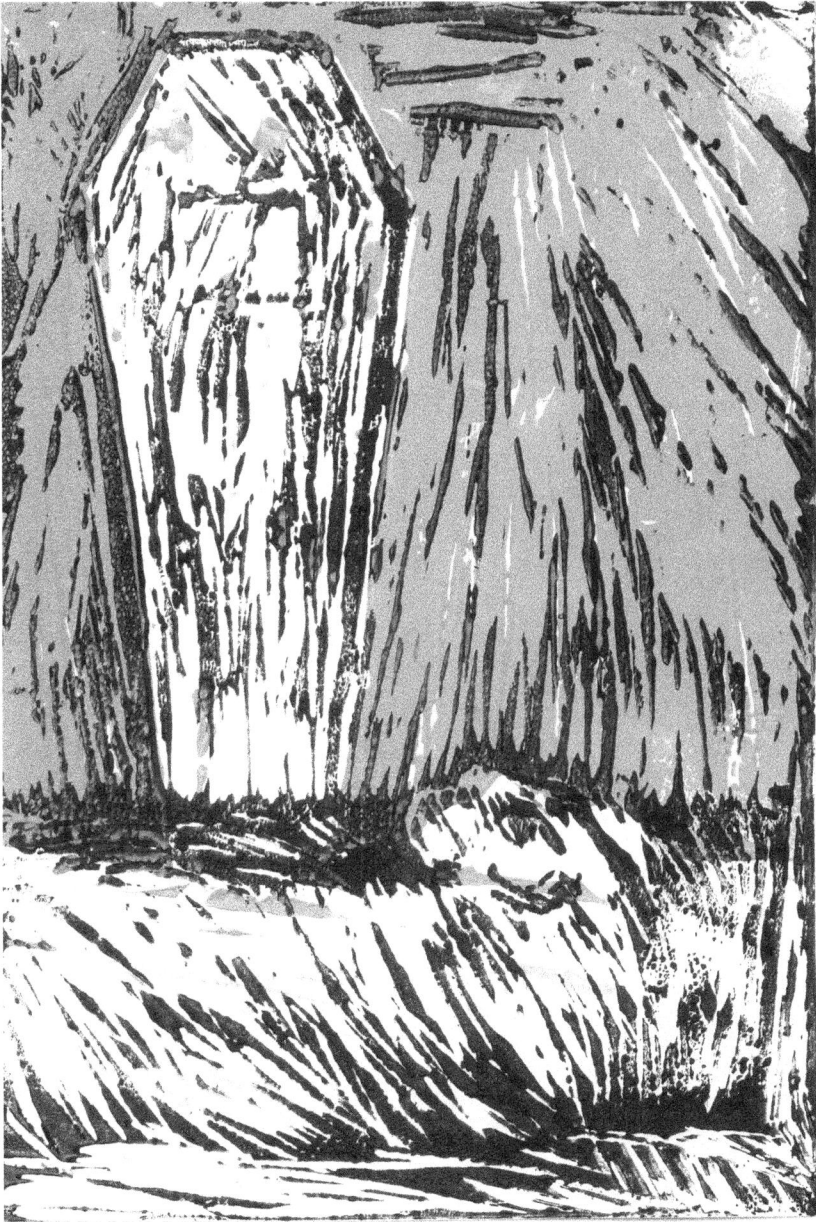

Figure 8.6 The Post Room-object Space. Lino Cut Print by D. Wright.

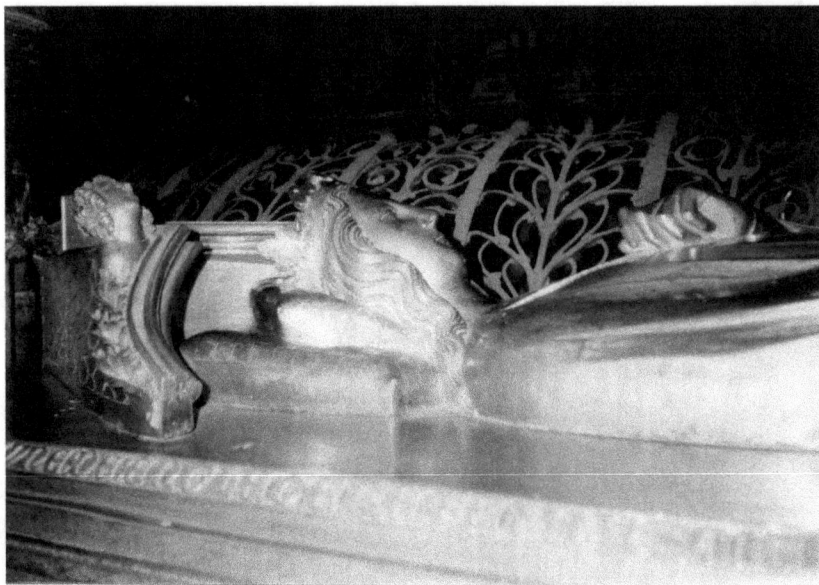

Figure 8.7 The Tomb of Eleanor of Castille, The Post Room-object space. Photograph by D. Wright.

embalmed body was sent on a procession from Lincoln to Westminster Abbey, through the area of her properties, and memorial crosses were erected at each night stay along the way such as 'Charing Cross' (the nearest to Westminster Abbey). She had triple *Post Room-object* spaces. Her organs (removed during embalming) were buried at Lincoln, her heart in the Dominican priory at Blackfriars in London, and her body was buried at Westminster Abbey in a tomb with a beautiful gilt-bronze effigy of her, that operates as Kantorowicz describes, preserving the decaying body inside as a split of deadness, the effigy, the split off part that lives forever preserves the memory and representation off her as alive and un-interfered with/threatened attached by the decaying body that shows the reality. As discussed, although this Post Room-object space (as well as the other 2 two Post-object spaces in Lincoln and Blackfriars as well as the spatial array of the procession and erection of crosses to mark out the spatial array) was created by King Edward to fulfil the public spatialising needs, and provoke object usage of her in this Post-Object-space space, we can say that she may have expected this and something of her own perfection to Post-death Post-death could be present there.

Freud was inspired by Eleanor's spatial array of what I am calling *Post Room-object* spaces, as we saw in Chapter 2 (see page 31) where he thinks of the Charing Cross sight (from the spatialised event of Queen Eleanor's burial processions): 'The monuments and memorials with which large cities are adorned are also mnemic symbols. [...] [W]hat should we think of a Londoner who paused today in deep melancholy before the memorial of Queen Eleanor's funeral [...] Not only do they remember painful experiences of the remote past, but they still cling to them emotionally (Freud, 1957[1910], pp. 16–17). Freud writes of placing these memorials on mourning path like 'Queen Eleanor') which he utilises as exemplifications of mnemic symbols; objects in space, into which feelings are not only projected but which are, in turn, constitutive of these feelings in the first place which here are a part of *Post Room-object* space.

Clinical Examples of Post Room-object; Ms G and Mr A

Ms G (Chapter 6) struggled to make a *Stage 5* space to have her Virtual Consulting room sessions during the initial period of the Virtual Consulting room, as in her new partner's flat there was nowhere that felt comfortable and safe enough, despite putting up the large Canvas photograph (itself a type of monument) of her mother, on the wall of the bedroom where she had some video-call sessions from. When she and her partner switched to living in her house and she created a study in her spare room, it was aided by her mum having slept in the bed which was then imbued with meaning and existed as a monument to her mum having spent time there. The room represented, simultaneously, a *Post Room-object* space as well as an enabling through meaningful link with her Mother a *Stage 2, 3 4,* and 5 space including mother.

Mr A (Chapter 1) showed me the photographs of his grandad just after his death as a memorial to him and thinking about him whilst looking at photos on screenshare with me. We could say I became the observer, seeing this space, just as the pilgrims in Westminster Abbey did when viewing the effigy of Queen Eleanor, as it was and what it represented. In addition, whilst looking at the photographs, Mr A found estate agent photographs on the internet, of his Grandad's house from when Mr A was young, and explored that this was a space of continuity and order after his mother and father broke up. This was a memorial to granddad but also to the original *Room-objects* space during the creating of a Stage 5 space via the Virtual consulting room. The Photograph, in Fig. 8.8 shows The Crusaders Tomb, in Westminster Abbey, which I have included at the end here as an interesting juxtaposition of imagery in the way that the composition of the photograph of the effigy, although split off from the real body, underneath, as Kantorowicz discussed, appears to be lying in wait to launch down the birthing passage; here represented by the space or 'body' of the Abbey in the distance, with a vagina-like end, through which life might begin again at any moment- this adds to the post room-object effect here.

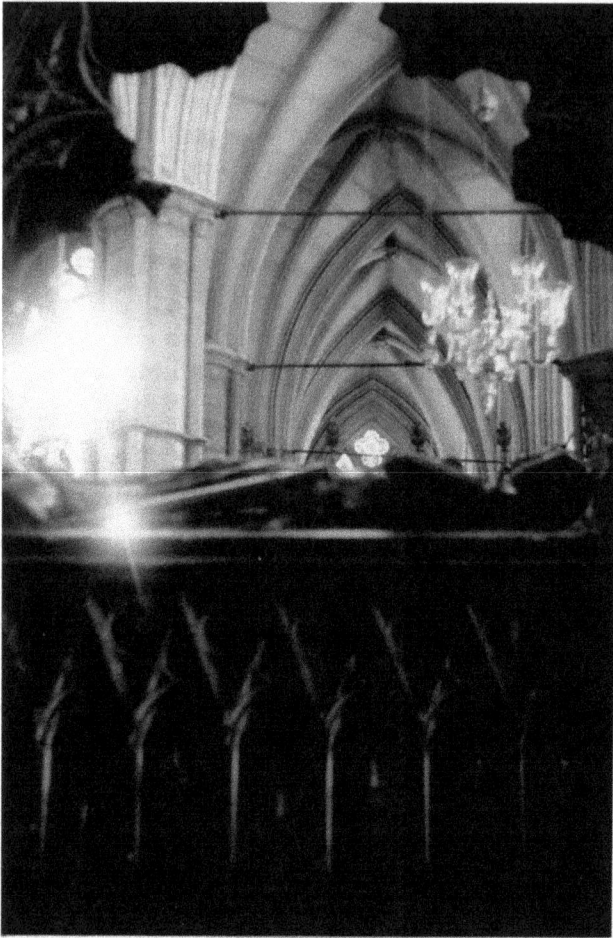

Figure 8.8 Crusaders Tomb, Westminster Abbey. Photograph by D. Wright.

The End Space Thoughts

At the end of his first book, *Aphasia a Critical Study*, Freud (1891) concludes:

> I have endeavoured to demolish a convenient and attractive theory of the aphasias, and having succeeded in this, I have been able to put into its place something less obvious and less complete. I only hope that the theory I have proposed will do more justice to the facts and will expose the real difficulties better than the one I have rejected. It is with

a clear exposition of the problems that the elucidation of a scientific subject begins.

(Freud, 1953 [1891], p. 104)

Freud is highlighting the attractiveness of concepts that conceal a lack of knowledge. Sweeping statements sometimes don't fit the phenomena and the evidence. In the case of Aphasia, it was localization. In the case I have explored, it is that everything in the room is transference. I have provided evidence of my formulation of the Room-object Spatial Matrix stages, in particular demonstrating the pre-transferential aspects. I can, therefore, conclude that I have established that there is a non-transferential component, which clears the way for presenting spatialisation as an ingredient of object relations. In addition, the evidence of the pre-object, pre-transferential aspects, makes way for the existence of the *Stage 3 – Consulting Room-object*. This is because the *Stage 1 – Primal Spatialisation* pre-object stage, can be spatialised into rooms *Stage 2 Room-object* and secondary spatialised into the consulting room (*Stage 3*), where at times, the consulting room functions as the stage 2, original spatialising room did, separate from any transference to the therapist. I am suggesting that there is a projection onto the room, not via the therapist, which is separate. I suggest that evidence of spatialisation (where instead of thinking actions occur in space) into rooms by Freud has not been taken up in psychoanalytic theory, perhaps because it was so personal and habitual for Freud and perhaps not entirely conscious. Then later generations, in identification with Freud, repeat his retaining of spatialisation in an unconscious or minimally conscious state. Freud's consulting room, the original psychoanalytic consulting room – was also Freud's *End Room-object space*, and we could also think of it therefore as *Post Room-object space* relating to Freud's original Room-object space.

Freud's fascination with the development of the mind included his attempt to find the original spatialisation, which creates the object world and is retained in transferences. I suggest that the *Stages 2–5* of the Room-object Spatial Matrix, are a defence against the feelings of the original *Stage 1 – Primal Spatialising* experience where spatialisation creates the original object through spatialising parts of mother. I suggest that this spatialising can be a lifetime pursuit (to be retreated in to as a defence) of re-constituting/re-creating/re-building the object mother to defend against the object's loss, or it getting damaged by anger/rage at its inadequacy. My formulations open up this subject for more investigation. I hope this does more justice to the phenomena in the physical space and the virtual space of the consulting room than the view that everything in the room is transference.

Henri Rey writes, 'Every time someone uses language to formulate a thought or to communicated it to others, he engages in a process of construction. [...] A process of non-verbal construction goes on simultaneously along with verbal activity. [...] In order to understand a message, the recipient has to analyse the message into bits and units of information, and to reconstruct the message for himself.' (Rey, 1994, p. 137). Patients are constructing communications, with themselves, the room, and the therapist all of the time from bits of verbal activity, non-verbal spatialising, and these can be moved in and out of through the stages of the Room-object Spatial Matrix as has been shown. Just like the original spatialised room (*Stage 2, Room-object*) offered top-up/replacement of the object/mother function, the role of the consulting room and the Virtual consulting room can be to provide top-up/replacement of the therapist function (separate to the transference to the therapist), depending on the need and ability to utilise the therapist in the transference, through an auxiliary space that can be related to by the patient transferentially and pre-object, pre-transferentially.

Figure References

Figure 8.1: In the ending room, the re-spatialised early bad room space, (Stage 1 of the Room-object Spatial Matrix) – Primal Spatialising. Lino-cut Print by D. Wright.

Figure 8.2: The End Room-object. Drawing by D. Wright.

Figure 8.3: Sigmund Freud's Consulting Room from the front – 20 Maresfield Gardens. Drawing by D. Wright.

Figure 8.4: The Couch upon which Sigmund Freud spent his final days and on which he died. Photograph © Freud Museum London.

Figure 8.5: Engraving by Adrien Moreau from the title page of Honoré de Balzac's The Magic Skin (1897) Philadelphia: George Barrie & Son, 1897. ile:BalzacMagicSkin01.jpg Created: 19th-century date QS:P,+1850-0000T00:00:00Z/7. https://en.wikipedia.org/wiki/La_Peau_de_chagrin#/media/File:BalzacMagicSkin01.jpg

Figure 8.6: The Post Room-object Space. Lino-cut Print by D. Wright.

Figure 8.7: The Tomb of Eleanor of Castille, The Post Room-object space. Photograph by D. Wright.

Figure 8.8: Crusaders Tomb, Westminster Abbey, Photograph by D. Wright.

References

Balzac, H. D. (1977) *The Wild Ass's Skin (La Peau de Chagrin)* (Trans Herbert J. Hunt), London, Penguin.

Freud, S. (1953 [1891] *On Aphasia A Critical Study*, Trans. And Intro E. Stengel, New York: International Universities Press.

Freud, S. (1957 [1910]) Five Lectures on Psycho-analysis. Tr. & ed. James Strachey *et al. Standard Edition of the Complete Psychological Works of Sigmund Freud*, vol XI. London: Hogarth Press and the Institute of Psychoanalysis. 1–56.

Gide, A. 1987 (1957) [Translated by Dorothy Bussy] [first published in France 1920 & first public addition 1924] *If It Die...* Harmondsworth: Penguin.

Jones, E. (1967 [1953]) *The Life and Work of Sigmund Freud.* Harmondsworth: Penguin.

Kantorowicz, E. H. (1957, repr. 1997) *The King's Two Bodies, A Study in Mediaeval Political Theology.* Princeton New Jersey: Princeton University Press.

Lacan, J. (2002 [1966]) *Ecrits* (Trans Bruce Fink in Collaboration with Heloise Fink and Russel Grigg). New York & London: W. W. Norton & Company

Leavitt D. (2005) Introduction *in* Forster E.M. (2005[1971]) *Maurice*, London: Penguin.

Rey, H. (1994) Universals of Psychoanalysis in the Treatment of Borderline and Psychotic States: Factors of Space-Time and Language. London: Free Association Books.

Segal, N. (1998) *Andre Gide: Pederasty and Pedagogy*, Oxford: Oxford University Press.

Steiner J. (1994) Foreword in *Universals of psychoanalysis in the treatment of psychotic and borderline states: Factors of Space-Time and Language* by Henri Rey (1994). London: Free Association Books.

Wright, D. (2018) Rooms as Replacements for People: The Consulting Room as a Room Object (pp. 251–262). In: *On Replacement – Cultural, Social and Psychological Representations.* Editors: Owen, J. and Segal, N., Switzerland: Palgrave Macmillan.

Index

Note: Page numbers in *italics* indicate illustrations.

For Product Safety Concerns and Information please contact our EU
representative GPSR@taylorandfrancis.com
Taylor & Francis Verlag GmbH, Kaufingerstraße 24, 80331 München, Germany

www.ingramcontent.com/pod-product-compliance
Lightning Source LLC
Chambersburg PA
CBHW060257220326
41598CB00027B/4136